# Microarrays for the Neurosciences

**Cellular and Molecular Neuroscience**

Charles F. Stevens, editor

# Microarrays for the Neurosciences:
# An Essential Guide

*edited by Daniel H. Geschwind and Jeffrey P. Gregg*

APPLIED BIOSYSTEMS

*A Bradford Book*
*The MIT Press*
*Cambridge, Massachusetts*
*London, England*

This book was set in Melior and Helvetica on 3B2 by Asco Typesetters, Hong Kong and was printed and bound in the United States of America.

Library of Congress Cataloging-in-Publication Data

Microarrays for the neurosciences : an essential guide / Daniel H. Geschwind and Jeffrey P. Gregg, editors.
    p. ;   cm. — (Cellular and molecular neuroscience)
 ''A Bradford book.''
 Includes bibliographical references and index.
 ISBN 0-262-07229-7 (hc.: alk. paper).
 1. Neurosciences. 2. DNA microarrays. 3. Gene expression. I. Geschwind, Daniel
H. Gregg, Jeffrey P. III. Cellular and molecular neuroscience series.
[DNLM: 1. Nervous System Physiology. 2. Oligonucleotide Array Sequence
Analysis—methods. 3. Gene Expression Profiling. 4. Nervous System Diseases—
genetics. WL 102 M626 2002]
RC343 .M46   2002
612.8—dc21                                                    2001056283

This book is dedicated to the memory of a great father and scientist, Stanley Geschwind. I thank my wife, Sandy, and three children, Eli, Maya, and Jonah, for their patience and love.

— DG

# Contents

# *Foreword*

We are just entering a dramatically new period in the biological sciences, the postgenomic era. As additional complete—or nearly complete—genomes become available, we have the possibility of determining which genes are active, and how active, in a variety of experimental circumstances and disease states in different organisms. This new potential for examining the role for expression of many genes in any context depends on knowing the sequences of all of the genes, the output of the genome projects, and on being able to detect gene expression, the job of the gene chips described in this book.

Although we all believe that DNA microarrays will revolutionize neurobiology, we do not have much idea of exactly how; at the outset of any new era, the course of the future is largely a delightful surprise. Many of us used to believe that the complexity of the brain arose from the "fact" that the majority of our genes are brain-specific. We now know that humans have many fewer genes than expected, and that brain complexity will have to arise out of patterns of gene expression rather than from the use of many brain-specific genes. We can be thus sure that many neurobiology laboratories will need to use gene chip analysis, and this book describes how to do it.

Charles F. Stevens

# *Preface*

Over the past several years there has been an explosion in biological information. This has been fueled by the exhaustive efforts of the Human Genome Project and private industry to sequence the human genome, the mouse genome, and the *Drosophila* genome, as well as the genomes of a number of model organisms and bacteria (Celniker, 2000; Collins and Mansoura, 2001). This unprecedented undertaking has generated a new discipline termed "functional genomics," or the study of the relationship of the genetic code and its biological potential. This staggering and complex amount of information and its associated biological relevance is quite unlike the traditional simplified analysis encompassing the study of one gene and one gene function. We now have the opportunity to observe the function of the predicted 30,000 human genes and determine their biological function—not on an individual basis, but globally (Lander et al., 2001; Venter et al., 2001). The ability to monitor the human genome (and other genomes) is due not only to our decoding of it, but also has been influenced by the development of sophisticated equipment and technology.

One of the first core technologies that has been utilized in genomics (after the automated sequencer) is DNA microarray technology for the study of gene expression (Schena, 1996; Lockhart and Winzeler, 2000). DNA microarrays represent one of the many areas where molecular genetics and genomics are revolutionizing neuroscience. Why all the excitement? Rather than looking at one gene at a time, DNA microarray technology offers the unprecedented ability to monitor the expression patterns of large numbers of genes simultaneously; this makes it relevant to almost every aspect of neuroscience research, including anatomy and physiology.

Classically, neuroscientists have often been divided into systems neurobiologists and molecular neurobiologists—two groups with little in common. One exciting aspect of the microarray revolution is that it offers the potential to elevate molecular genetic approaches for studying the nervous system to the systems level.

Using DNA microarrays to monitor the expression of thousands of genes simultaneously requires a more macro or large-scale view of the system being studied. As microarray studies become more common and technical details become less pressing concerns, methods for data reduction and modeling will become the prominent themes in the application of this technology. These are areas where systems neuroscientists and physiologists tend to be stronger than the molecular neurobiologists.

To us, the most interesting phenomenon is the intersection, or clash, of the genomics paradigm with neuroscience. Typically, neuroscience has looked askance at "fishing expeditions," while genetics has thrived on "screening." The most state-of-the-art modern neuroscience has been focused on detailed functional studies of single molecules, and usually has not been descriptive. Despite each of their biases, both the genetics and neuroscience paradigms have been remarkably successful. Now in an era where almost every human gene has been identified, the application of genetic screening methods to the problems in which neuroscientists are most interested will likely reap great rewards. One recent example of this is the study of brain tissue from deceased schizophrenic patients to identify a potentially unifying molecular theme in this disease (Hakak et al., 2001; Mirnics et al., 2000).

In this book we begin to explore DNA microarrays, emphasizing topics of relevance to the neuroscientist and tackling the unique aspects and challenges that the nervous system poses for this new discipline. We believe this is the first book on microarrays written with a central nervous system (CNS) theme.

The genesis of this book stems from a short course on microarrays in which we were involved at the Society for Neuroscience meeting in Miami, Florida, in 1999. Prior to the meeting, one of us had published a paper on looking at gene copy number by using microarrays (Geschwind et al., 1998a) and had one of the few abstracts on the use of microarrays at the meeting (Geschwind et al., 1998b). Based on this small body of work, he was asked by the society's Education Committee to organize a short course on the topic, focused on the concerns of the neuroscientist. Although other fields, particularly cancer biology, had rapidly adopted arrays, neuroscience was more hesitant. We do not think that this was an inappropriate oversight or demonstrated ignorance of a powerful new technology, but rather was a reflection of the caution of investigators who appreciated the complexity of the nervous system relative to other organs or model systems.

In contrast to the study of the CNS, the disciplines of yeast, cell, and cancer biology have the luxury of having biological systems that are more easily adaptable to gene expression studies. These systems are much less complex, usually involve one cell type, and obtaining abundant appropriate material for studying gene expression is relatively simple and inexpensive. For example, many cancers are believed to be clonal expansions of a single cell type that has undergone an incipient genetic mutation. Therefore, the comparison of the parental cell (normal) with the expanded clonal neoplastic population is built on the fact that the two populations are more alike than they are different; a single (or perhaps a few) genetic insult has caused a catastrophic change in the cell behavior, but the initial genetic complexity of the system is relatively small.

The CNS has the most cellular heterogeneity and tissue complexity, and it is believed that most of the predicted 30,000 human genes will be expressed at some level in the CNS, whereas only a small subset will be expressed in any particular somatic tissue. However, the CNS poses more difficult challenges than just number of genes and amount of data. The number of cell types, the architecture, the developmental program, and the importance of environmental factors in CNS development and functioning are unprecedented in their contribution to CNS tissue complexity. Do

changes in gene expression reflect alterations in tissue composition, rather than changes in gene expression by a particular cell
type (e.g., Eberwine et al., 1992)? Furthermore, the presence of
many different types of cells in a single small piece of tissue may
limit the microarray detection of low-abundance RNAs that are of
interest (Geschwind, 2000). In addition, on a very practical level,
the CNS network being studied may involve small anatomical
regions with only a few thousands of cells, and the ability to obtain
these samples poses additional challenges (Eberwine et al., 1992;
Emmert-Buck et al., 1996).

Cell lines, which are the staple of other disciplines, are often
considered too simple, and not representative of the true in vivo
behavior of neurons and glia. Processes discovered or studied in
neuronal or glial cell lines usually have to be confirmed in vivo or
in tissue culture so as to be most convincing. All of these issues
pose significant challenges for the study of comprehensive gene
expression in the brain and nervous system.

This book focuses on the neuroscientist and includes specific
chapters that address these prominent obstacles. We have assembled a group of individuals who have each approached their area
of expertise with care and considerable thought.

We begin with a basic technical introduction to the key aspects
of the methodology. In the first chapter, Dr. Gregg gives a broad
overview of the technology platforms for gene expression studies,
including a discussion of equipment and resources. In the next
chapter, Dr. Pickett and colleagues provide a detailed discussion of
array scanning and image acquisition, followed by Drs. Shah and
Shams, who consider the complex issues of image and data analysis. Dr. Nadon and colleagues then give a broad but elegant discussion of the statistical methods needed for array analysis.

The next group of chapters discusses specific applications of
gene expression studies in the CNS, each with its unique perspective and technology. Dr. Becker and colleagues discuss the benefits
of using membrane arrays to study gene expression and provide
detailed descriptions of the methods this group has used to profile

gene expression in neurologic disease. Rather than using the typical two-color fluorescent hybridization, they use radioactively labeled probes, enabling the use of small starting RNA quantities with high sensitivity of detection. Dr. Becker therefore demonstrates that the membrane arrays provide a tried-and-true platform that one can adapt without new equipment and large expense.

Dr. Chiang and colleagues then take us through a strategy of informatically and experimentally selecting genes enriched in the nervous system for inclusion onto arrays, rather than blindly purchasing a commercial array simply because it is available. This ensures that genes of interest will be studied. With proper design, the information content of each array can be very high and contain very few irrelevant data points. Dr. Chiang also uses radioactive probes on membrane arrays, further demonstrating the utility of this approach described by Dr. Becker. Protocols and websites with updates are provided to enable the readers to adapt this technology in their laboratories.

In the next chapter by Dr. Awad and colleagues, the focus changes to the GeneChip, an oligonucleotide platform developed by Affymetrix. This chapter provides a complete overview of oligonucleotide technology. In addition, several applications of this technology are discussed, including the study of regional and strain-specific variation in gene expression in the mouse brain. This kind of basic information on strain and regional differences will be an important foundation from which future experimentation will benefit greatly. It highlights the need for centralized repositories of expression data so that other investigators can make maximal use of this important resource (Becker, 2001; Geschwind, 2001). But, despite its clear benefits, controversy over data sharing remains (Miles, 2001; Mirnics, 2001).

Postmortem human tissue is an important source of material for the study of human neuropsychiatric disease. Its use raises many issues, including the need to control for genetic heterogeneity and postmortem artifacts. The chapter by Dr. Van Deerlin and colleagues provides a detailed summary of the issues and strategies to be considered when using human postmortem tissue. It also discusses RNA amplification from small samples and is an invaluable resource in this regard. Dr. Potier and colleagues describe one powerful approach to limiting cellular heterogeneity by discussing different strategies for microdissection and isolating single cells for further gene expression analysis. By isolating a defined region or cell type that has been studied electrophysiologically, they systematically decrease the complexity and minimize the extraneous "noise" other cell types may contribute. This further allows elegant genotype–phenotype functional correlation on a single-cell level.

The applications portion of the book finishes with a chapter by Drs. Geschwind and Nelson, describing the strategy of using cDNA subtraction coupled to the microarray to identify differentially expressed genes. This strategy offers the ability to quickly collate groups of differentially expressed genes that include novel or previously unsuspected genes. This novel strategy benefits from letting the biology select the important genes, rather than relying on theoretically predefined clone sets or arrays. It also allows for novel gene discovery in addition to gene expression analysis. This chapter also emphasizes the need to follow up on some of these array screening experiments with expression studies such as *in situ* hybridization.

In the future, analytic approaches will gain center stage as the technology becomes more widely used and more data are generated. The field of microarray data analysis is in its infancy, and as an example of its potential, we conclude with a chapter by Dr. Fuhrman and colleagues that describes novel methods using microarray data to develop hypotheses about regulatory networks.

Where possible, websites are included to permit more in-depth exploration of the methods and resources available. We have also included our current protocols where possible so as to facilitate any of these experiments in the reader's laboratory. It is our hope that this book gives individuals that have never performed an array experiment the excitement and energy to apply this technology to their own studies. For the more experienced microarray enthusiast, we hope that we have provided the tools to help perform a better microarray experiment. We urge our fellow neuroscientists to adopt this technology, and have a chip on their bench, rather than on their shoulder.

# References

Becker KG (2001). The sharing of cDNA microarray data. *Nature Reviews/Neuroscience* 2: 438–440.

Celniker SE (2000). The drosophila genome. *Curr Opin Genet Dev* 10: 612–6.

Collins FS and Mansoura MK (2001). The Human Genome Project. *Cancer* 91: 221–5.

Eberwine J, Yeh H, Miyashiro K, Cao Y, Nair S, Finnell R, Zettel M, and Coleman P (1992). Analysis of gene expression in single live neurons. *Proc Natl Acad Sci USA* 89: 3010–14.

Emmert-Buck MR, Bonner RF, Smith PD, Chuaqui RF, Zhuang Z, Goldstein SR, Weiss RA, and Liotta LA (1996). Laser capture microdissection. *Science* 274: 998–1001.

Geschwind DH (2001). Sharing gene expression data: An array of options. *Nature Reviews/Neuroscience* 2: 435–438.

Geschwind DH (2000). Mice, microarrays, and the genetic diversity of the brain. *Proc Natl Acad Sci USA* 97: 10676–8.

Geschwind DH, Gregg J, Boone K, Karrim J, Pawlikowska-Haddal A, Rao E, Ellison J, Ciccodicola A, D'Urso M, Woods R, et al. (1998a). Klinefelter's syndrome as a model of anomalous cerebral laterality: Testing gene dosage in the X chromosome pseudoautosomal region using a DNA microarray. *Dev Genet* 23: 215–29.

Geschwind DH, Loginov M, Karrim J, Nelson SF (1998b). Finding the differences between the developing cerebral hemispheres using RDA and DNA microarray technology. *Society for Neuroscience Abstracts* 24(1): 398.3

Hakak Y, Walker JR, Li C, Wong WH, Davis KL, Buxbaum JD, Haroutunian V, Fienberg AA (2001). Genome-wide expression analysis reveals dysregulation of myelination-related genes in chronic schizophrenia. *Proc Natl Acad Sci USA* 98(8): 4746–51.

Lander ES, Linton LM, Birren B, Nusbaum C, Zody MC, Baldwin J, Devon K, Dewar K, et al. (2001). Initial sequencing and analysis of the human genome. *Nature* 409(6822): 860–921.

Lockhart DJ and Winzeler EA (2000). Genomics, gene expression and DNA arrays. *Nature* 405: 827–36.

Miles MF (2001). Microarrays: Lost in a storm of data. *Nature Reviews/Neuroscience* 2: 441–443.

Mirnics K (2001). Microarrays in brain research: The good, the bad and the ugly. *Nature Reviews/Neuroscience* 2: 444–447.

Mirnics K, Middleton FA, Marquez A, Lewis DA, and Levitt P (2000). Molecular characterization of schizophrenia viewed by microarray analysis of gene expression in prefrontal cortex. *Neuron* 28: 53–67.

Schena M (1996). Genome analysis with gene expression microarrays. *Bioessays* 18: 427–31.

Venter JC, Adams MD, Myers EW, Li PW, Mural RJ, Sutton GG, Smith HO, Yandell M, et al. (2001). The sequence of the human genome. *Science* 291(5507): 1304–51.

# *Microarrays for the Neurosciences*

# 1 Microarrays: An Overview

*Jeffrey P. Gregg*

Microarrays can be defined as DNA attached to a solid substrate in an ordered manner at high density. Typically, oligonucleotides or amplified cDNA inserts (representing expressed sequences or genes) are attached to a solid surface. Hundreds to thousands of these products can be immobilized on a very small area with a specialized robotic arraying apparatus. The immobilized products (i.e., the array) serve as hybridization targets for a labeled probe. This probe is generated by extracting RNA and labeling it with fluorescence, radioactivity, or chemiluminescence. The labeled probe is then hybridized to the array and a high-resolution image is created using a specialized scanner. Software is then used to determine the intensity of each spot and to calculate statistics and confidence intervals. Finally, the processed data can be analyzed in order to see patterns or associations between genes and samples. See figure 1.1 for a detailed description.

In real terms, DNA microarrays provide an indispensable platform that offers the ability to analyze extremely large amounts of information in a massively parallel fashion. Arrays are relatively simple; they can be made inexpensively (in terms of the amount of data generated); and they provide a versatile tool for a diverse number of applications, including the assessment of the expression of genes, querying the genetic code at the level of a single base pair, and determining DNA copy number or ploidy.

Over the past few years, interest in microarrays has been growing exponentially. This unabashed enthusiasm has been elevated by the announcement of the sequencing of the fruit fly genome (Adams et al., 2000), the completion of sequencing of the human

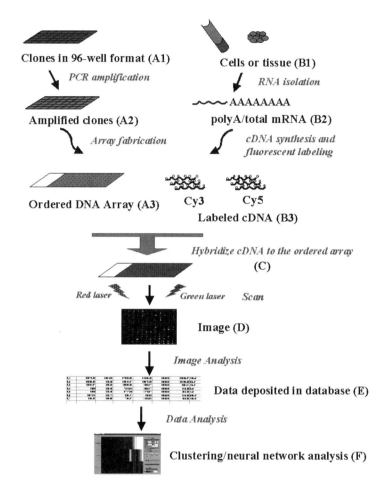

**Figure 1.1** Overview of the cDNA microarray process.

genome (Lander et al., 2001; Venter et al., 2001), and the anticipated completion of the sequencing of the mouse genome. In addition, we are coming to the realization that full genome expression profiles are distinctly possible in the near future.

Yet, despite the scientific community's enthusiasm for the widespread use of array technology, the field is still relatively young. One of the first forays into array technology was by Brown's laboratory at Stanford University (Schena et al., 1995). This was one of the first laboratories to develop an in-house integrated microarray system and it has set up a website that provides instructions on how to build a scanner and arrayer, as well as numerous protocols for experimental application (http://cmgm.stanford.edu/pbrown/mguide/index.html).

DeRisi, at the University of California, San Francisco, was one of the many individuals in the Brown laboratory who was instrumental in developing array technology (DeRisi et al., 1997; Lashkari et al., 1997). His website provides additional information that is especially suited to the academic or "do-it-yourself" user (http://www.microarrays.org).

The infrastructure and high-throughput nature of array technology makes it particularly suitable for an integrated pharmacogenomics approach. Affymetrix, as well as Molecular Dynamics (now Amersham Pharmacia Biotech [AP Biotech]), Incyte Genomics, and Hyseq, have filled this niche and offer integrated microarray systems. Recently, Agilent Technologies (in collaboration with Rosetta Inpharmatics) has entered this high-end market.

The cost of a fully integrated microarray system is substantial, and such systems are generally inaccessible to the individual research program. However, by now most universities and the National Institutes of Health have come to the rescue and have invested significant sums of capital to build microarray cores with some of these high-end technologies. In addition, some of the companies have reduced array prices significantly for academic users. Therefore, with the availability of equipment and lower array prices, the use of these technologies is not unrealistic for individual researchers, although it is still very expensive.

The great danger now lies in performing poorly controlled and statistically invalid experiments because of the prohibitive expense of performing multiple replicates. Perhaps the most realistic application of array technology for the academic researcher over the next few years will be to use these high-end vendors, or off-the-shelf arrays, for an initial comprehensive analysis of many genes (full genome) with a few screening experiments. The differentially expressed subset of genes obtained from the initial experiments then can be validated with many more experiments with less expensive technology, providing statistically significant results and findings.

The enormous increase in the number of manufacturers of arrayers, scanners, slides for spotting, and other array-related equipment over the past several years can be overwhelming for a researcher trying to enter the microarray field. The goal of this chapter is to give the reader a summary of array technology by briefly discussing some of the current technologies and providing an overview of companies that are producing array-related products. Because the microarray field is highly dynamic and rapidly changing, the list of companies and technologies discussed here is not all inclusive, but I have tried to incorporate as much relevant information as possible. In addition, new information about array companies and products is updated on the websites listed in the appendix. Several general microarray protocols are provided at the end of this chapter.

It is the aim of this chapter to provide information on how to obtain the appropriate resources for developing a microarray system, whether it be for doing a first array or for setting up a core resource in an academic laboratory. Ultimately, I hope this chapter gives the reader a better understanding of arrays and provides sufficient background facts to help researchers make informed decisions about array instrumentation and methodologies.

### Arraying Formats

There are two basic types of arraying formats: (1) oligonucleotide arrays (15–25 base pairs), and (2) spotted arrays that contain larger DNA fragments generated by polymerase chain reactions (PCR), genomic clones (100 base pairs or greater), or large oligonucleotides (50–75 base pairs).

In general, oligonucleotide arrays are created by attaching hundreds to thousands of short oligonucleotides (15–25 base pairs) to a solid support either by directly synthesizing the oligonucleotide onto the surface or by chemically attaching column-synthesized oligonucleotides to a solid support. In chapter 7 Awad and colleagues describe this process in detail. Arrays created using the former format are now commercially available. Affymetrix is one company that produces oligonucleotide arrays in this fashion (Pease et al., 1994; Chee et al., 1996), and they have substantially increased their core products (GeneChips) for gene expression in the human, mouse, and rat, and recently also for single-nucleotide polymorphisms (SNPs). In the gene expression area, each array can contain from a few hundred to about 15,000 data points.

Historically, one of the general limitations of these arrays has been that they cannot be easily changed or customized for expression analysis. Therefore the researcher was limited to using the preformatted arrays that are available or waiting months to obtain a smaller custom array. Affymetrix has addressed this by beginning to produce custom arrays of 1000 genes, culled from genes found on the larger arrays per the investigator's instructions. The cost of these arrays ranges from about $250 to $1000 per GeneChip or about $0.10–0.50 per data point (gene expression values). Agilent Technologies (a spinoff from Hewlett-Packard) has just entered the array market and utilizes its parent company's ink-jet technology to deposit either oligonucleotides or amplified cDNA inserts onto a solid surface. This technology promises to be very powerful, so that the researcher may be able to individually select the genes of interest and print them onto the custom array. The true setup costs for these custom array services should be substantially less than those for custom GeneChips.

In contrast to oligonucleotide arrays, spotted DNA arrays can be made relatively inexpensively (less than $100 per 10,000 array when made in batches) and provide flexibility in construction to fit the individual researcher's interests. These spotted microarrays are created by coupling DNA fragments (PCR products, genomic clones, large oligonucleotides) to a solid surface via ultraviolet (UV) irradiation, covalent chemical bonds, or baking.

## Arrayers

With regard to arrayers, the first decision to make is whether to construct your own arrayer or buy a pre-made commercial arrayer. A parts list and detailed instructions for constructing an arrayer can be found on the Brown laboratory website, but even with this valuable resource, one should expect a significant amount of time in addition to material costs (which are equivalent to the cost of the lower-end commercially available arrayers). On the other hand, commercial manufacturers of arrayers provide a finished product and service that includes customer and technical support. Therefore, for laboratories that wish to rapidly begin arraying, it is more efficient to purchase a commercial arrayer.

There are at least nine companies producing commercially available arrayers (see the appendices at the end of this volume). The essential component of all the systems is the spotting mechanism. There are four different types of spotting technologies: quill-based, modified replicating tool, Pin-and-Ring, and piezoelectric.

The first arrayer, developed by Brown's group, utilized a quill-based tip (figure 1.2). In this format, the tip is dipped into the DNA solution and the DNA is drawn into the quill through capillary action. About 1 µl or less is drawn into the tip. The tip is then tapped onto the glass slide (using a mechanical robot), depositing a small amount of DNA solution (about 0.5–1.0 nl). One major advantage of these tips is their ability to produce very small spots,

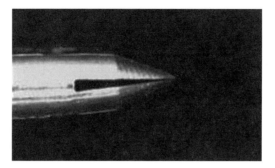

**Figure 1.2** Quill-based pin. Notice the pinched-in tip needed to create small spots.

and therefore high-density arrays can be made. The number of spots per standard $1 \times 3$-inch slide can approach 30,000.

However, the construction of the quill tip is difficult and necessitates engineering expertise. The quill needs to be fashioned to deposit a small amount of fluid consistently, which is difficult since some tips inherently produce large spots while others may not deposit any liquid at all. This is a key issue because in order to increase the speed of producing high-density arrays, up to 64 quill tips can be used together. It is essential that these tips produce similar spots, but producing sets of tips that behave similarly has been troublesome. In academic centers, machine shops have been used to fashion these tips with variable results. Therefore, alternatives have emerged. TeleChem International, Inc. is a company that manufactures quill tips that generally produce small, consistent spots. These tips can be ordered singly or in matched sets, and each tip costs about \$200–\$300.

In addition to the spot consistency problems, one of the major drawbacks of the quill-based tip has been its propensity to clog with DNA or salt solutions. With a clogged tip, no DNA is deposited, which can be disastrous for an individual generating a large array. This inherent problem has created the need to constantly monitor the spotting in order to catch and clean clogged tips. For this reason, the ability to automate these systems has been limited. However, automation is now becoming more robust with better tip design and improved tip-washing protocols. Some systems have incorporated a sonication station to mitigate the tip clogging.

A new opportunity in this type of technology has emerged with AP Biotech's decision to sell its DNA spotter individually rather than as an inclusive package (previously requiring purchase of the spotter, arrayer, and access fee). This spotter is priced competitively, produces high-quality arrays in a high-throughput fashion, and seems to have overcome many of the problems associated with quill tips.

The second type of arrayer is based on a solid pin, or modified replicating tool. In general, these pins produce poor-quality arrays, and they inconsistently spot onto glass, although they have the advantage of spotting well onto membranes. In chapter 6 Chiang and colleagues provide a powerful argument for the use of high-density spotted membranes using solid pins. However, most researchers who plan on using only glass arrays will abandon this pin type owing to its poor performance unless they plan to also use membrane arrays.

The Pin-and-Ring system designed by Genetic Microsystems (now Affymetrix) is a unique system that utilizes a ring that is dipped into the DNA solution. The ring captures about 1 µl of liquid via surface tension (much like dipping a loop into a soapy solution for blowing bubbles). A needle then penetrates the meniscus, capturing a very precise amount of fluid on its tip. The tip is then touched to the surface of the slide, depositing the fluid (figure 1.3 and plate 1).

The advantage of this system is that a very consistent amount of fluid is deposited with each spotting. The spots are consistent within and between tips (each Pin-and-Ring). In addition, there is a much lower risk of tip clogging than there is with the quill-based system. Furthermore, these tips can also be used to create high-density membrane filter arrays in addition to glass arrays. However, the Pin-and-Ring system cannot match the density of the quill-based array systems because of the current physical constraints on the size of the pins.

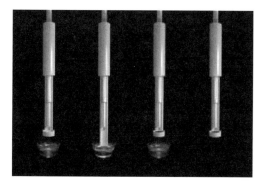 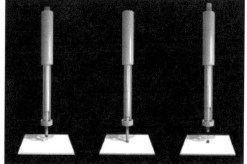

**Figure 1.3**  Pin-and-Ring system from Affymetrix (formerly Genetic Microsystems). See plate 1 for color version.

Another essential aspect of arrayer systems using pins is the robot that controls the positioning and spotting mechanisms of the pins. In general, there are two types of robots: (1) machines that have been modified from colony pickers and (2) robots that have been designed specifically for arraying onto glass and membranes. The modified robots, including those from BioRobotics, Genetix, and Beckman, generally have the most robust features for automating the arraying process. These features include plate-handling capacity, lid lifting, and bar coding. In addition, they generally can produce more arrayed slides per run, and the speed of arraying is quite fast.

The main disadvantage of these systems is that in the past, the arraying heads have had poor position accuracy in spotting arrays. However, many companies are addressing this issue, and spotting accuracy is improving. The array-specific robots (Cartesian, Gene-Machines, Affymetrix [GMS], Genomic Solutions, and AP Biotech) have very high position accuracy and therefore can produce very dense arrays. Each of these companies is upgrading its accessories (or has already done so) to include plate-handling capability and bar coding for increased automation, and some are going to include environmental controls (humidity, temperature, air filters). For the most current product and technology information, refer to the individual manufacturer's website (see the web resource list at the end of this volume).

The software to run each of these robots is evolving rapidly. Most of the software packages are limited and need improvement, but it is expected that all the major suppliers of arrayers will gradually upgrade their software to meet the needs of the customer.

Finally, there is the piezoelectric technology for arraying. In these systems, the DNA is sprayed onto the array much like ink is sprayed in ink-jet printers. This technology is exciting, but there remain many technical problems that have limited its use. These problems include the inability to spray viscous DNA solutions, clogging of the jets, high void volumes, and inefficient cleaning of jets between DNA samples. Piezoelectric technology has been most successful in applying oligonucleotides to solid surfaces rather than larger PCR fragments. However, this technology is quickly becoming more reliable and efficient, and it is likely that we will be seeing better systems very soon. Agilent Technologies is one of the first companies to commercially produce arrays with this technology, and the initial results look promising.

**Scanners**

The second major piece of equipment needed to set up an array core is the high-resolution fluorescent scanner, although for filter arrays using radioactivity (described in chapter 5 by Becker and colleagues), this equipment is not necessary. As with arrayers, the early investigators engineered and built their own scanners (Shalon et al., 1996). However, scanners have proven to be more technically challenging to build than the arrayers because of the expertise needed in engineering, optics, and computer programming. Owing to these difficulties and the rapid emergence of technically sound commercial scanners, the majority of the microarray pioneers have now purchased commercial units.

The increased numbers of scanner manufacturers and the continual development of new and improved designs of existing models have made the field extremely dynamic. There is a wide range of differences among scanners, ranging from the scanning mechanism, to cost, to software. Thus, comparing scanners is difficult, with the major challenge being the ability to assess sensitivity and dynamic range of signal detection. A comprehensive and fair side-by-side comparison of all the systems has not been performed or published, yet rumors abound, with outlandish claims of scanner performance (generally not from the manufacturers, but from individual researchers). The following paragraphs discuss the important aspects of the scanners and compare and contrast the systems where it is possible. In chapter 2 Pickett and colleagues provide more background on the technical considerations involved in scanning. Current scanner information can be found on the manufacturers' websites (see the list at the end of this volume).

In simplistic terms, there are two scanning mechanisms for array-based imaging: (1) the charge-coupled device (CCD) camera and (2) the laser. The laser systems are the predominant design and include the models from Packard Biochip Technologies (Packard Bioscience, Inc.), Affymetrix (Genetic Microsystems), Virtek Vision International, AP Biotech (Molecular Dynamics), Beecher Instruments, Axon Instruments, and Agilent Technologies.

The first versions of these scanner systems provided the ability to detect two nearly nonoverlapping fluorescence emission spectra —550 and 649 nm—corresponding to the emission of the fluorescent dyes Cy3 and Cy5 (AP Biotech). These two fluorescent dyes have been the reagent of choice for nearly all laboratories producing fluorescent microarrays. They are particularly suitable because they have nonoverlapping spectra and the lasers used for excitation are relatively cheap and small (e.g., fluorescein needs an argon laser that has to be externally cooled). In addition, other companies have been slow to develop alternative dyes. Currently, there are number of Cy3 alternatives (550 nm), but it has been difficult to find a substitute for Cy5 (649 nm). Therefore the Cy dyes have been incorporated into almost all protocols and into popular microarray culture. This has been unfortunate, since Cy5 is less stable and also seems to incorporate into cDNA less efficiently than does Cy3, leading to a potential dye bias that complicates experiments. In addition, the cost of the dyes is high, although Perkin Elmer Life Sciences (formerly NEN Life Sciences) now offers equivalent Cy3 and Cy5 dyes. In the spirit of capitalism, this competition between manufacturers has begun to reduce the prices of dyes. Some new fluorescent labeling technologies (to be discussed later in this chapter) that have been developed also offer some alternatives to the traditional dyes and dye incorporation protocols.

More recently, the ability to image a wider variety of dyes has emerged. This has been made possible by adding additional lasers to laser-based systems or different filter selections in CCD camera-based systems. Virtek and Packard Bioscience have four- and five-laser systems. For practical reasons, few laboratories are currently using more than two colors, since the prices on these four-laser models are fairly high, and there are few array-based software packages and limited data on dye combinations for the additional dyes.

Although it may be an attractive option to add the ability to scan a third color as a quantification control, the benefit of adding other dyes and spectra needs to be balanced with price and the ability to fully utilize such a machine. Based on current prices of the $4^+$-color units ($> \$100,000$), it would seem prudent to purchase a more affordable two-color system and rely on patience until the practicality and price of the $4^+$-color units become more reasonable.

The speed of scanning is an issue with the laser-based systems. The machine from Axon Instruments has the fastest scanner in the laser-based arena. It essentially scans and captures the Cy3 and Cy5 signals simultaneously. The Affymetrix instrument is a bit slower than the Axon instrument, and the speed of scanning for the new models from Packard Bioscience approaches that of the Affymetrix scanner. On the slower machines, it may take as long as 5 to 10 minutes per color to scan an entire slide ($1 \times 3$ inches), whereas it takes only about 2 to 3 minutes to complete a two-color scan of the same slide on the Axon instrument. This becomes a throughput issue as the number of arrays and number of colors to be read increases. To the anxious researcher, the faster scan speed of the Axon machine may have advantages. In addition, several of the machines (e.g., AP Biotech, Agilent Technologies, Affymetrix) now have automated slide loading and scanning capability, and this can be a key feature for high-throughput laboratories.

The performance parameters of CCD-based machines are still a bit unknown. The machines are limited to imaging small areas, making them difficult to use in scanning the large areas needed for microarrays. Applied Precision Imaging (API) has developed a system that can mesh many small captured areas into a single frame, thus depicting the entire slide. Using this new technology development, API has released their first commercial scanner. It uses a single white light for excitation and therefore offers flexibility in the fluorescent spectra it can analyze. This may be a feature needed for individuals creating and evaluating new dyes and gives the researcher the flexibility to use an assortment of different wavelength dyes. However, the processing power needed to weave the images together is considerable. The images are also very large, initially making them impractical for the standard desktop computer. However, advances in computer chip technology now permit this system to be operated by a standard desktop CPU.

For microarray applications, it is essential to have a scanner with high resolution. This has been one of the main features of all the new scanners. Traditional flat-bed scanners have a resolution of 50–100 µm, whereas most of the array-based scanners have a resolution of 10 µm (each pixel is 10 by 10 µm). This resolution is more than adequate for the analysis of arrays with a density of up to 10,000 facets per square centimeter. For higher-density arrays, some of the newer machines have 5 µm resolution. The image files for these high-resolution scans can become quite large, with an entire scan area occupying about 10–20 MB per color.

One of the most important benchmarks for scanners is their sensitivity and dynamic range. In reality, most of the scanners compare favorably, and claims of dramatic differences in sensitivity and dynamic range are probably misinformed. As mentioned earlier, there have been no definitive side-by-side tests of the latest machines from individual companies in order to make qualified judgments. In addition, each company makes almost monthly improvements, so that the comparisons done today may be invalid a month later.

As the scanner market has increased in the number of manufacturers, it seems that three companies—Packard Bioscience, Affymetrix, and Axon Instruments—have taken most of the market share; Agilent Technologies has just entered the market and may become a major player. A detailed analysis of all of these machines is lacking, and the instruments are not available to compare side by side owing to long waiting lists for purchase and high consumer demand for demonstrations.

In terms of software, Axon Instruments and Packard Bioscience have developed their own internal software for data analysis. In addition, with the purchase of an Axon scanner, three site licenses for the imaging software are provided. This is a useful feature because array image processing can be time-consuming, and having several sites gives a laboratory the ability to have multiple users on different computers.

Affymetrix is developing software that will offer communication between their arrayer and scanner, enabling the scanner to know the position and identity of all arrayed facets. This is another desirable feature, since it can also be time-consuming to populate gene expression databases with clone identity. In addition, BioDiscovery, Inc. produces niche software for the array market, including a user-friendly and elegant package called ImaGene for data acquisition, analysis, and visualization. BioDiscovery also produces a package called CloneTracker that can interact with a number of different arrayers and populate the gene expression data fields with the correct clone identification, gene ID, and names. Both of these packages can be used on any scanner platform. More up-to-date information about array software can be found on the developers' websites.

An additional factor, which may need to be addressed, is the use of hydrated slides in scanning. Cy3 and Cy5 are scanned dry without a cover slip, but other dyes need to be hydrated and have a cover slip applied in order to maximize their intensity (e.g., the Alexa dyes and phycoerythrin from Molecular Probes, Inc.). If use of one of these alternative dyes is required or foreseen to be required in the future, the choice of scanner for the laboratory may need to be adjusted. In addition, the cover slip changes the focal point, so the focus for the confocal scanners will need to be adjusted. With some of the instruments this adjustment may be trivial, while with others it may be impossible.

**Slides**

Our group has performed detailed comparisons of slide manufacturers and conditions for producing the best arrays. As with arrayer and scanner manufacturers, companies making "microarray" slides are emerging in the marketplace daily. Due to the rapid change in technology, we suggest checking websites and microarray user groups (e.g., Gene-Arrays@ITSSRV1.ucsf.edu) to obtain more up-to-date information. We have evaluated some of the more prominent brands and suppliers. Initially, we investigated different surface coatings of glass slides [aminoalkylsilane coated, poly-L-lysine coated, and 1,4-phenylene diisothiocyanate derivatized (PDC)] to attempt to maximize DNA coupling to the surface. Both amino-modified and nonamino-modified PCR-amplified target products were tested. In addition, we evaluated buffer solutions for resuspension of the target DNA using a concentration titration series of sodium citrate (SSC) and sodium bicarbonate buffers. Attachment of the DNA for the poly-L-lysine and silanated glass slides involved UV irradiation (see the protocol at the end of this chapter).

Silanated glass slides gave the highest signal intensity and the most reproducible DNA attachment, while maintaining the lowest background fluorescence. The poly-L-lysine slides produced lower signal and high background fluorescence in our hands. In the buffer series, 350 mM sodium bicarbonate buffer (pH 9.0) allowed the highest hybridization signal on the silanated glass slides. The amino-modified PCR products produced a decrease in signal compared with the nonamino-modified products in the silanated slides using the sodium bicarbonate buffer and an insignificant signal change in the SSC series.

In recent tests, the silanated CMT–GAPS slides from Corning produced very high signal and very low background. These slides are very expensive, up to $12/slide, but these high costs are well worth the expense if high-quality data are produced. TeleChem International also produces a number of slides that are made in a very rigorous fashion. These are expected to provide high-quality data as well, although they have not yet been tested in our laboratory. Sigma is now making microarray-specific slides that should be of high quality, but again, they have not yet been tested in our laboratory. However, the general immunohistochemistry "silane-prep" slides from Sigma were, in our hands, very inconsistent for microarray purposes. By the time this volume is published, more vendors, such as NEN, will also have released commercial slides.

For optimal attachment, the DNA concentration to be arrayed is as important as the slide surface. This concentration should be at least 200 ng/μl, with optimal performance occurring with concentrations above 400 ng/μl. With the Affymetrix arrayer, concentrations of 750 to 1000 ng/μl produce a greater signal, whereas concentrations below 250 ng/μl produce a very poor signal. In short, the message is that it is better to err on the side of having too much DNA rather than too little, but in most protocols, concentrations greater than 400 ng/μl produce excellent results.

## Signal Amplification Reagents

There are two new reagents that can potentially increase signal and decrease the amount of starting RNA needed for slide-based array experiments. The first is the 3DNA technology from Genisphere.

In this format, total RNA is reverse transcribed by poly-deoxy-thymidine (dT) priming. In this step, no fluorescent nucleotide is incorporated; thus there is efficient cDNA synthesis.

This can be contrasted with the very inefficient incorporation of Cy dye-labeled deoxycytidine triphosphate (dCTP) or deoxy-uridine triphosphate (dUTP) in the direct labeling procedures that most laboratories use. The fluorescent dyes are large and bulky and the reverse transcriptase tends to stutter and slow when it encounters the dyes. The enzyme tends to stall, producing short or incompletely labeled cDNAs.

The novel aspect of the Genisphere 3DNA technology is that the poly-dT primer also includes an added nucleotide capture sequence; this sequence binds to a complementary DNA sequence attached to the 3DNA fluorescent probes. Each probe carries an average of 250 Cy dye molecules. Therefore the cDNA is synthesized more efficiently and each cDNA is labeled with the equivalent of 250 Cy dyes. In this format, it is possible to use 10–50-fold less RNA (250 ng to 25 µg of total RNA) with equivalent or better sensitivity than traditional direct incorporation. Further, the 3DNA labeling protocol is relatively simple.

However, although the manufacturer has shown that this reagent has a high degree of reproducibility, achieving this level of reproducibility in individual laboratories may take considerable effort on the part of the researcher. An additional disadvantage is the expense of the product, but this must be considered in the context of the benefit of small sample size.

Another exciting technology that is now commercially available is an optimized kit for tyramide substrate amplification and fluorescent detection (TSA, Perkin Elmer Life Sciences). This type of kit has been used in immunohistochemistry amplifications with success; preliminary experiments by beta testers (Karsten et al., 2002) attest to its relatively high reproducibility. The method is more time-consuming than the 3DNA protocol, but has actually been easier to adapt to individual laboratories thus far. Further, the cost is lower, thus making it a reasonable alternative for signal amplification.

## Prearrayed Slides

Over the past year, there has been a dramatic increase in the number of manufacturers of prearrayed slides. They have ranged from low-density (or very niche-oriented arrays) to high-density arrays. One of the earliest commercial array makers was Clontech, Inc. (now BD Biosciences), which has significant experience in manufacturing membrane arrays. They have several membrane arrays commercially available, and they now sell a 1024-facet glass array. The unique aspect of BD Biosciences' system is that the user receives a labeling cocktail that includes a set of multiplexed primers specific for each gene on the array. Therefore the complexity of the labeling product is theoretically simplified by increasing the sensitivity and specificity of hybridization.

Invitrogen (Research Genetics) produces high-density GeneFilter membrane microarrays, including multiple releases of human, rat, and mouse libraries. In addition, they are one of the distributors of the IMAGE clone sets and now offer ready-made PCR products for spotting onto arrays.

Perkin Elmer Life Sciences produces a prearrayed system, which incorporates its tyramide amplification reagents and protocols with prearrayed slides. This system, like the BD Biosciences system, benefits from including both the labeling technology and prearrayed slides.

Corning, the maker of CMT–GAPS slides, attempted to enter the commercial array market but has since discontinued its commercial prefabricated arrays. The first arrays it produced included a full yeast genome array and a 6000–10,000 facet human array. One of the benefits of these commercial prearrayed slides compared with independent, academically created arrays is the ability of these array makers to include significant quality assurance protocols. For example, Corning had sequence-verified all of its clones and then subsequently sequence-verified all the PCR products to be arrayed. For the academic laboratory, this is unfeasible in cost and time. Unfortunately, the cost of the prearrayed slides is also fairly high at this time and most academic researchers will be forced to create their own arrays. The most current information on the availability and pricing of premade arrays can be found at the manufacturers' websites.

## Conclusion

This chapter has attempted to outline some of the infrastructure that is needed for developing a laboratory with microarray capabilities or core resources. In the following chapters, you will be exposed to the cutting edge of array technology, methods, and informatics. Special attention should be paid to the themes of RNA amplification and the informatics approaches to storing, processing, and analyzing array data.

The complexity of the nervous system is unmatched by any other physiological system; therefore, there is going to be a need to reduce this complexity by using very anatomically defined portions of the nervous system or pure populations of cells. This will require the use of very small amounts of material and sometimes single-cell analysis. In addition, the complexity of expression profiles in the nervous system is going to demand novel and robust computational tools in order to understand the relationships and biology. Good luck and enjoy the journey.

**Protocol 1:** PCR amplification of target DNA for arraying

- The quantity of Taq polymerase used must be optimized for the type of Taq used, and may have to be optimized for each library being used as template.
- In order to ensure spots of the highest quality, the minimum quantity of product in each well must be greater than 5 µg for arraying. If necessary, do multiple PCR reactions and pool the products in one plate to obtain the minimum yield.
- PCR reactions must be carried out in a 96-well format. Final products for arraying must be in skirtless polycarbonate plates (Costar catalog #6509).

**Necessary reagents per reaction**

PCR

10 μl 10× PCR buffer (100 mM Tris-HCl, 300 mM KCl, 100 mM $(NH_4)_2SO_4$,
   15 mM $MgCl_2$, 0.1% Triton X-100)
2 μl 10 mM dNTPs
2 μl 10 μM forward primer
2 μl 10 μM reverse primer
0.8–1.0 μl Taq polymerase
2 μl template culture
$ddH_2O$ up to 100 μl

ETHANOL PRECIPITATION

5 μl 3 M NaOAc
70 μl cold 100% EtOH
100 μl cold 75% EtOH

**PCR procedure**

1.  Make a master mix of all reagents except the template and put into a sterile
    reagent reservoir (keep on ice).
2.  Using a multichannel pipettor, aliquot 98 μl of the master mix to each well.
3.  Using a multichannel pipettor, aliquot 2 μl of culture with the desired insert
    to each well, mixing gently.
4.  Cycle in thermal cycler under the following conditions:

| STEP | TEMP (°C) | TIME | NO. OF CYCLES |
|---|---|---|---|
| Denaturation | 96 | 3 min | 1 |
| Denaturation | 94 | 30 sec | |
| Annealing | Depends on primer $T_m$ | 30 sec | 35 |
| Extension | 72 | 90 sec | |
| Extension | 72 | 5 min | 1 |
| Hold | 4 | Indefinitely | — |

5.  Check 5 μl of each sample on a 1.5% agarose gel for presence of insert.
6.  The bands obtained should be of a quality and intensity similar to those in
    this sample gel:

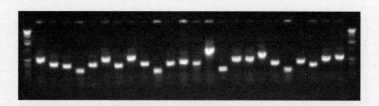

7. Dry down samples so that the volume in each well is ~50 μl. Samples may be heated at 50 °C for this step.

**Ethanol precipitation**

1. Make a master mix of 3 M NaOAc and 100% EtOH.
2. Using a multichannel pipettor, aliquot 75 μl of master mix to each well.
3. Seal plate with plastic sealer and incubate overnight at −20 °C.
4. Spin at 4 °C for 1 hour at >3000× *g*.
5. Decant supernatant and wash pellets with 100 μl of 75% EtOH.
6. Spin at 4 °C for 30 minutes at >3000× *g*.
7. Decant supernatant and dry pellets.

**PCR product resuspension**

1. If it is necessary to pool reactions, resuspend products well (by alternately vortexing and spinning) in sterile filtered ddH₂O and pool in one plate. Dry down clones before resuspending in arraying buffer.
2. When ready to array, resuspend products well by vortexing and spinning in at least 12 μl of desired filtered arraying buffer (such as 350 mM sodium bicarbonate, pH 9.0, with 0.1% sarcosyl).
3. If arraying >24 hours after resuspension of PCR product, dessication of the sample may have occurred; it is necessary to dry down the clones and resuspend as described below.
4. If products have been previously resuspended in buffer, they can be reused by resuspending well in >12 μl of filtered ddH₂O.

**Protocol 2:** Direct incorporation of fluorescent nucleotides during reverse transcription

- Make sure to take measures to minimize any possible RNase contamination when handling mRNA.

- Execute all steps involving fluorescent nucleotides in as dimly lit an environment as possible. Perform all lengthy incubations in the dark.

**Necessary reagents per reaction**

0.5–2.0 µg polyA mRNA (resuspended in 14.5 µl of ddH$_2$O)
2.0 µl 1 µg/µl oligo dT 21-mer
1.0 µl dNTP cocktail (12.5 mM dATP, dGTP, dTTP; 7.0 mM dCTP)
0.5 µl RNase block (Stratagene catalog #300151)
1.0 µl Cy3 dCTP (Amersham catalog #53021)
1.0 µl Cy5 dCTP (Amersham catalog #55021)
5.0 µl 5× SuperScript II (SSII) first-strand buffer (Gibco/BRL catalog #18057-018)
2.0 µl 200 U/µl SSII reverse transcriptase (RT) (Gibco/BRL catalog #18064-014)
Microcon-30 spin column assembly (Millipore catalog #42409)

**Procedure**

1. Combine polyA RNA and oligo dT 21-mer and denature at 65 °C for 5 minutes.
2. Anneal at room temperature for 10 minutes.
3. Add the following:

   CY3 LABELING
   5.0 µl 5× SSII buffer
   1.0 µl dNTP cocktail
   0.5 µl RNase block
   1.0 µl Cy3 dCTP
   1.0 µl SSII RT

   CY5 LABELING
   5.0 µl 5× SSII buffer
   1.0 µl dNTP cocktail
   0.5 µl RNase block
   1.0 µl Cy5 dCTP
   1.0 µl SSII RT
4. Mix gently and incubate at 42 °C in the dark for 1 hour.
5. Add an additional 1.0 µl SSII and incubate for another hour in the dark at 42 °C.
6. Put on ice to stop reaction, spin down, and pool Cy3 and Cy5 reactions.
7. Add 5 µl 10 mM EDTA to stop the reaction.
8. Add 5 µl 0.5 M NaOH to hydrolyze residual RNA.

9. Incubate at 65 °C in the dark for 10 minutes.
10. Add 25 µl 1 M Tris HCl, pH 7.5 to neutralize the solution.
11. Pre-rinse the Microcon-30 unit with 2× 500 µl sterile ddH$_2$O.
12. Apply the labeling reaction to the Microcon-30 unit. Rinse the sample tube with 100 µl sterile ddH$_2$O and add to labeling reaction.
13. Spin at 14,000 rpm in microcentrifuge for 6 minutes, or until volume is concentrated to about 50 µl.
14. Invert Microcon-30 unit in a fresh collection tube and spin at 3500 rpm for 3 minutes.
15. Speed-vac probe to dryness (in dark).
16. Resuspend dried probe as described in hybridization protocol (protocol 4).

**Protocol 3:** Random labeling of cDNA/PCR products with fluorescent nucleotides

- Execute all steps involving fluorescent nucleotides in as dimly lit an environment as possible. Perform all lengthy incubations in the dark.
- As an alternative to ethanol precipitation of the labeled probe, one can run the sample through a MicroSpin S-200 column (Amersham Pharmacia Biotech #27-5120-01) following the manufacturer's general protocol. The sample will then need to be dried down in a lightproof speed-vac.

**Necessary reagents per reaction**

1.0–2.0 µg cDNA or PCR product (resuspended in 22.5 µl of ddH$_2$O)
10.0 µl 27 OD/ml random 9-mer primers
1.6 µl 2.5 mM dA/T/G mix (2.5 mM each of dATP, dTTP, and dGTP)
2.0 µl 250 µM dCTP
2.0 µl Cy3 or Cy5 dCTP (Amersham catalog #53021 or #55021)
5.0 µl 10× random priming buffer
2.0 µl 5 U/µl exo(-) Klenow fragment polymerase
10 µl 3 M NaOAc
200 µl cold 100% EtOH
200 µl cold 75% EtOH

**Procedure**

1. Combine DNA and 9-mer primers and denature at 95 °C for 5 minutes.
2. Place on ice slurry until cool, spin down, and place on ice again.
3. Add the following:

CY3 LABELING
10.0 µl 10× random priming buffer
1.6 µl dATG
2.0 µl dCTP
2.0 µl Cy3 dCTP
2.0 µl exo(-) Klenow

CY5 LABELING
10.0 µl 10× random priming buffer
1.6 µl dATG mix
2.0 µl dCTP
2.0 µl Cy5 dCTP
2.0 µl exo(-) Klenow

4. Mix gently and incubate at 37 °C in the dark for 4–12 hours.
5. Put on ice to stop reaction, spin down, and pool Cy3 and Cy5 reactions.
6. Add:
   5.0 µl 0.5 M NaOH
   5.0 µl 10 mM EDTA
7. Incubate at 65 °C in the dark for 10 minutes.
8. Add:
   10 µl 3 M NaOAc
   200 µl cold 100% EtOH
9. Precipitate labeled DNA at −20 °C overnight.
10. Spin samples at maximum speed in a microcentrifuge at 4 °C for 30 minutes.
11. Remove supernatant and wash pellet with 200 µl 75% EtOH.
12. Spin samples at maximum speed in a microcentrifuge at 4 °C for 10 minutes.
13. Remove supernatant and allow pellets to air dry (in dark).

**Blocking agent solution (makes enough solution for 20 hybridizations)**

INGREDIENTS

$C_0 t$-1 DNA(Gibco/BRL)
Poly(dA) (Amersham-Pharmacia)
Yeast RNA (supplied with $5' \rightarrow 3'$ Northern buffers)
3 M NaOAc
Cold 100% EtOH
Cold 75% EtOH
Sterile ddH$_2$O

FINAL CONCENTRATIONS

5 μg/μl $C_0t$-1 DNA
4 μg/μl Poly(dA)
2.5 μg/μl Yeast RNA

**Procedure**

1. Resuspend poly(dA) to 1 μg/μl.
2. In a 1.5-ml tube, mix together:
   220 μl 1 μg/μl $C_0t$-1 DNA
   176 μl 1 μg/μl poly(dA)
   5.5 μl 20 μg/μl yeast RNA
   Note: quantities assume 10% loss of yield during precipitation steps.
3. Add: 40.2 μl 3 M NaOAc
   803 μl cold 100% EtOH
4. Precipitate overnight at −20 °C.
5. Pellet precipitate by centrifuging at maximum speed in microcentrifuge at 4 °C for 30 minutes.
6. Discard supernatant and wash pellet with 1 ml cold 75% EtOH.
7. Spin at maximum speed in microcentrifuge at 4 °C for 10 minutes.
8. Air dry pellet.
9. Resuspend in 40 μl sterile $ddH_2O$.
10. Store at −20 °C.

**Protocol 4:** Hybridization of labeled probe to cDNA array

**Postarray slide preparation**
For slide preparation procedures, use only pre-prepared 95% ethanol (we use Fisher catalog #NC9585277). Do not prepare 95% ethanol from 100% ethanol (residual denaturants from the manufacture of 100% ethanol may interfere with subsequent hybridization and/or scanning).

NECESSARY REAGENTS

0.1% Sodium dodecylsulfate (SDS) (room temperature)
$H_2O$ (room temperature)
$H_2O$ (95 °C)
95% EtOH (ice cold)

NECESSARY EQUIPMENT

Heat block set to 95 °C
Stratalinker (Stratagene)
Coplin jars
Lantern slide racks (Shandon-Lipshaw #144)
Plate carriers
Centrifuge equipped with sealed microtiter

**Procedure**

1. Hydrate slides (face down) over a beaker of steaming water for several seconds until moisture is evident on array surface.
2. Snap-dry slides (face up) on a 95 °C heat block for several seconds until all evidence of moisture is gone from the array surface.
3. Place slides in Stratalinker and UV cross-link at 400 mJ (4000 μJ × 100).
4. Place slides in Coplin jar with 0.1% SDS and incubate for 1 minute.
5. Rinse slides in Coplin jar with room temperature $H_2O$.
6. Place slides in Coplin jar with 95 °C $H_2O$ and incubate for 1 minute.
7. Place slides in Coplin jar with ice-cold 95% EtOH and incubate for 1 minute.
8. Remove slides from Coplin jar, place in balanced slide racks, and spin dry at low speed in centrifuge.
9. Store slides in dust-free box until ready for use.

**Prehybridization**
Depending on the size of the cover slip you use, the amount of prehybridization solution you need will vary. A 22 × 22-mm cover slip will use 10–12 μl of solution. A 22 × 40-mm cover slip will use 15–20 μl of solution.

**Necessary reagents and materials per array**

1× Prehybridization solution
2 μl blocking agent solution (see recipe above)
Hybrislip cover slip (Grace BioLabs)

**Procedure**

1. Combine desired quantity of prehybridization solution (see note) with 2 μl of blocking agent solution.
2. Heat solution to 95 °C for 5 minutes.
3. Apply solution to array and cover with Hybrislip.
4. Incubate array at 42 °C for 30–60 minutes.

**Hybridization**
Use the same amount of solution for hybridization as was used for the prehybridization.
When working with a fluorescently labeled probe, take care to minimize exposure of the sample to light.

**Necessary reagents and materials per array**

1× Hybridization solution
2 µl Blocking agent solution (see recipe above)
Hybrislip cover slip (Grace BioLabs)
Syringe and 18-gauge needle
Rubber cement

**Procedure**

1. Resuspend labeled probe pellet in appropriate volume of hybridization solution.
2. Add 2 µl blocking agent solution.
3. Heat solution to 95 °C for 5 minutes.
4. Apply solution to array and cover with Hybrislip.
5. Seal edges of Hybrislip with a generous amount of rubber cement (dispensed with syringe and needle).
6. Incubate array in the dark at 42 °C overnight (16–20 hours).
7. Wash array twice in wash buffer (3% SDS, 1 mM EDTA, 40 mM $Na_2PO_4$) for 5 minutes at room temperature with agitation.
8. Rinse array once in 0.2× SSC for 5 minutes at room temperature with agitation.
9. Spin array dry at <500× g.
10. Scan array at wavelengths appropriate for Cy3 and Cy5.

For other protocols see:

1. Brown Laboratory website (http://cmgm.stanford.edu/pbrown/protocols/index.html/)
2. microarrays.org (www.microarrays.org)
3. TIGR website (www.tigr.org/tdb.microarray)

# References

Adams MD, Celniker SE, Holt RA, Evans CA, Gocayne JD, Amanatides PG, Scherer SE, Li PW, et al. (2000). The genome sequence of *Drosophila melanogaster*. *Science* 287(5461): 2185–95.

Chee M, Yang R, Hubbell E, Berno A, Huang XC, Stern D, Winkler J, Lockhard DJ, Morris MS, and Foder SP (1996). Accessing genetic information with high-density DNA arrays. *Science* 274(5287): 610–14.

DeRisi JL, Iyer VR, and Brown PO (1997). Exploring the metabolic and genetic control of gene expression on a genomic scale. *Science* 278(5338): 680–6.

Karsten SL, Van Deerlin VMD, Sabatti C, Gill LH, Geschwind DH (2002). An evaluation of tyramide signal amplification and archived fixed and frozen tissue in microarray gene expression analysis. *Nucleic Acids Res* 30(2): in press.

Lander ES, Linton LM, Birren B, Nusbaum C, Zody MC, Baldwin J, Devon K, Dewar K, et al. (2001). Initial sequencing and analysis of the human genome. *Nature* 409(6822): 860–921.

Lashkari DA, DeRisi JL, McCusker JH, Namath AF, Gentile C, Hwang SY, Brown PO, and Davis RW (1997). Yeast microarrays for genome wide parallel genetic and gene expression analysis. *Proc Natl Acad Sci USA* 94(24): 13057–62.

Pease AC, Solas D, Sullivan EJ, Cronin MT, Holmes CP, and Foder SP (1994). Light-generated oligonucleotide arrays for rapid DNA sequence analysis. *Proc Natl Acad Sci USA* 91(11): 5022–6.

Schena M, Shalon D, Davis RW, and Brown PO (1995). Quantitative monitoring of gene expression patterns with a complimentary DNA microarray. *Science* 270(5235): 467–70.

Shalon D, Smith SJ, and Brown PO (1996). A DNA microarray system for analyzing complex DNA samples using two-color fluorescent probe hybridization. *Genome Res* 6(7): 639–45.

Venter JC, Adams MD, Myers EW, Li PW, Mural RJ, Sutton GG, Smith HO, Yandell M, et al. (2001). The sequence of the human genome. *Science* 291(5507): 1304–51.

## 2 *Microarray Scanning and Data Acquisition*

*Siobhan Pickett, Trent Basarsky, Damian Verdnik, and David Wellis*

The great promise of microarray technology is the possibility of determining the expression patterns and interrelationships of thousands of genes simultaneously (Botstein and Brown, 1999; Lander, 1999; Schena and Davis, 2000). However, the brightest spots and the most dramatic changes on a microarray may not necessarily indicate the genes that cause the most significant biological activity. Small changes in expression levels, and/or changes in the activity of low-expressing genes, can trigger significant cellular events. It can be extremely difficult to quantify such small changes.

To be confident that one has collected all the data worth having, one must have an objective measure of the quality of a microarray image.

- Microarray image quality can be quantified by the signal-to-noise ratio (SNR).
- Maximizing the signal-to-noise ratio maximizes the useful data that one can extract from a microarray.

When using fluorescent microarrays, changes in expression levels are measured as differences in the signal intensities from fluorescently labeled DNA ("labeled sample") hybridized to printed DNA samples ("printed sample") arrayed onto a glass support. For general reviews on the subject, see Bowtell, 1999; Brown and Botstein, 1999; Cheung et al., 1999; Schena, 1999. The fluorescent spots can be detected because they emit light in response to appropriate illumination. The emission that is derived from such fluorescence is known as the "signal."

The characteristics of the background affect the ability to detect and quantify arrayed spots (Basarsky et al., 2000; Zhou et al., 2000). High background levels obscure the signal from low-expressing genes, so that changes in expression may not be detected. In addition, the background is rarely a perfectly uniform field. These fluctuations in signal are called "noise." High background noise can impede accurate quantitation. There are many types and sources of noise that will be discussed later in this chapter, but regardless of the origin of the noise, it can typically be quantified by calculating the standard deviation of the background pixel values.

Once a signal has been separated from its background, it is straightforward to assess data quality by computing the signal-to-noise ratio:

$SNR = (\text{signal} - \text{background})/(\text{standard deviation of background})$

This calculation is commonly used in many signal-processing disciplines, including radio, electronics, and imaging. The SNR indicates the confidence with which a signal can be detected and quantified above the background noise. A commonly accepted criterion for the minimum signal that can be accurately quantified (i.e., the detection limit) is the sample value for which the signal is three times greater than the background noise:

$SNR = 3 = \text{detection limit}$

Below this point, features may be visible, but the ability to accurately quantify them diminishes (figure 2.1).

The best way to maximize the useful data from a fluorescent microarray is to maximize the SNR for all samples so that accurate data can be extracted from ever-lower expressing genes. The SNR can be optimized by increasing the signal measurement, decreasing the background, or decreasing the standard deviation (SD) of the background (figure 2.2).

The accuracy of the resulting data is ultimately determined by the cumulative contribution of each step in the process, including:

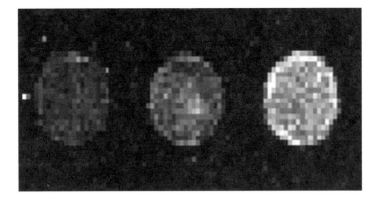

**Figure 2.1** A row of three microarray features with varying SNRs. The center feature has an SNR of approximately 5. Features with an SNR of less than 3 can still be seen, such as the dimmer feature to the left, which has an SNR of 1.3. The feature to the right has an SNR of 8.7.

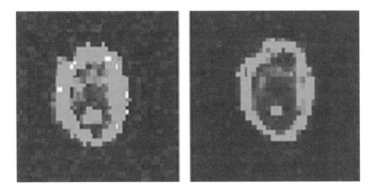

**Figure 2.2** The same features of a microarray scanned on two commercially available micro-array scanners. The feature on the left appears brighter than the feature on the right. However, the SNR of the feature on the left is about 40% less than the SNR of the feature on the right. The standard deviation of the background has reduced the SNR.

Array creation
Data acquisition (fluorescent excitation and signal collection)
Image generation
Data extraction
Results analysis

This chapter explains how each step of the microarray process can influence the SNR by affecting signal levels, background levels, and background noise. Taking steps to maximize the SNR improves the accuracy of the data and ultimately the confidence in interpretation of the results.

## Array Creation

One of the most common sources of background signal is the hybridized microarray sample itself. Utmost care must be taken to minimize all sources of background when creating fluorescent microarrays. In addition, the highest possible hybridization signal levels are ensured by proper care of all fluorescent reagents, and by optimizing DNA binding and hybridization conditions. Each of these steps can be optimized to maximize the SNR.

Glass microscope slides are commonly used as a convenient support matrix for microarrays created by mechanical deposition (for example, Botwell, 1999; Cheung et al., 1999; Schena, 2000). Other types of arrays are also available, and most of the issues discussed here apply to all fluorescent microarrays. Impurities in low-grade glass and coating reagents can fluoresce and increase both overall background signal and irregular noise. Nonuniform coating of the slide can cause irregular binding of the target, leading to low signal, and/or target loss. Nonuniform coating will also allow variable nonspecific DNA binding, thereby causing high and/or irregular background signal.

Most forms of DNA can be bound to appropriately coated glass slides. Polymerase chain reaction products and oligonucleotides are the most commonly used samples in mechanical deposition arrayers. Regardless of the DNA type, all samples must be carefully purified prior to arraying. Certain components in common biochemical buffers can inhibit arrayed DNA from binding to the glass. If the inhibition is such that the DNA in the arrayed spots is not in excess relative to the hybridized probe, the signal in the resulting hybridized spot may be low. If the fluorescent hybridizing probe is in excess, signal levels will not accurately represent the expression levels of the hybridized genes. In addition, the DNA binding capacity of glass is lower than that of commonly used blotting membranes, so there may be significant excess arrayed DNA at each spot (Piétu et al., 1996; Karpf et al., 1999).

Fluorescently labeled hybridizing samples must also be carefully purified after labeling. Unincorporated fluorescent nucleotides and short extension products can increase both background noise and overall background signal. Nonspecific hybridization can be minimized by optimizing the hybridization and the stringency of washing solutions and temperatures.

Fluorescent compounds absorb and emit light of different wavelengths with different efficiencies. For a review of fluorescence microscopy, see Rost, 1991. As indicated by their characteristic absorption and emission spectra, they absorb energy from a range of wavelengths. Excessive exposure to any light within the absorption spectrum, including white light, can cause photobleaching. The mechanisms of photobleaching are not completely understood, but Song and colleagues (1996) suggest that it is related to the accumulation of a long-lived triplet state involving destruction of the fluorochrome or changes in its quantum efficiency. All fluorescent components in a microarray experiment must be protected from light whenever it is practical during each phase of the experiment.

As with many biochemicals, repeated freeze-thaw cycles and unfavorable chemical conditions can also degrade fluorescently labeled nucleotides. To maximize signal by promoting efficient probe labeling and hybridization, fluorescent compounds should be protected from light, and the manufacturers' handling instructions should be followed exactly.

**Data Acquisition**

Although signal-to-noise considerations spread across sample preparation, data acquisition, and data extraction, the overall sensitivity of the hardware portion of this process should not be based on any single specification. It is necessary to consider the system as a whole or, in other words, as a tightly integrated group of components that work together. In this section, the various components of a microarray scanner are reviewed and consideration is given to how each may contribute to the overall SNR of the system.

The basics of microarray image acquisition are simple: Illuminate the microarray and collect the fluorescence emission. The trick is to send photons only where they need to be sent, to collect only the photons that are appropriately derived from the sample, and to accurately measure the collected photons.

**Light Delivery**

Earlier we presented an equation for the SNR. The signal ($S$) is related to the hardware in a number of ways. Very simply, $S$ is proportional to the number of photons ($N$) emitted from the sample, multiplied by the quantum efficiency ($QE$) of the detector. Quantum efficiency is the effectiveness of a detector in producing an electric charge from incident photons. We will address QE issues later in the discussion of detectors.

There are two general methods for illuminating or exciting fluorescent dye molecules on a microarray: broadband illumination and laser illumination (although light-emitting diodes could also be used). For general reviews, see Reichman, 1994, Booth and Hill, 1998, and Inoue and Spring, 1997.

Broadband illumination, or white light, is normally produced with an arc lamp, either mercury or xenon (the gases inside the lamp itself). Mercury and xenon lamps usually emit somewhere in the range of one hundred to a few hundred milliwatts of light, but this power measure is of the entire wide band. The lifetime of arc lamps is a few hundred hours at best and arc lamps are usually used for "flood" illumination in CCD-based systems. Mercury and xenon lamps emit very different profiles of white light, with the xenon bulb showing much more homogeneity across the spectrum.

All fluorescent molecules have an excitation spectrum, or range of wavelengths, that excites the dye. With broadband illumination, this white light must be filtered with an optical filter, or bandpass filter. The filter is chosen so that the light that illuminates the array overlaps the excitation spectrum of the dye of interest, but does not contaminate the emission spectrum of the dye. The almost unlimited supply of optical filters affords a broadband illumination source with great flexibility. However, the ultimate power delivered to the sample is not as high as that which can be obtained by laser illumination. Lower power means a longer collection time is required, which causes other problems—such as photobleaching—in attempting to optimize the system's SNR.

The absolute signal emitted from a sample depends upon the number of fluorescent molecules at the sample site, the dye's physical characteristics, and the power of the incident light. For dim spots on a microarray, the weak emission signal becomes more susceptible to photon noise within the light itself. For such low light-level scanning, the photon noise within the illumination varies according to the square root of the signal. Very low light-level signals have a relatively low signal-to-photon noise ratio. To maximize the emitted signal, fluorescence imaging instrumentation should apply the maximal illumination possible without photobleaching or extinguishing the dye. Photobleaching refers to the nonreversible decay in the efficiency of the dye in emitting photons, whereas extinguishing refers to reducing fluorescence by having too many fluorescent molecules emitting in a small area.

In contrast to arc lamps, laser illumination has a more limited choice of wavelength, and the power of some available wavelengths can be quite low. The advantage, however, is that a relatively high power of monochromatic light can be concentrated in a point of light delivered to the sample. Since the laser light can be more powerful than arc lamps at some wavelengths, less time is required to excite the fluorescent molecule. The most commonly used dyes for microarrays, such as the cyanine-based dyes (Amersham Pharmacia Biotech, Perkin Elmer Life Sciences), are excitable by available laser wavelengths.

Table 2.1 shows the lasers most commonly used for microarray and genomics research. Cy3 (Amersham Pharmacia Biotech), for example, can be excited by either a doubled yttrium-aluminum-garnet (YAG) laser with a wavelength of 532 nm or by a helium neon (HeNe) laser with a wavelength of 543 nm. Cy5 can be excited by a 635-nm diode laser or by a 633-nm HeNe laser. It is generally recommended that the optimal illumination be slightly shorter in wavelength than the peak of the excitation spectrum of the dye. Keeping the illumination shorter than the peak allows a broader band collection of the emitted light. In addition, the emitted light is less likely to be contaminated with laser light. The signal-(emitted light)-to-noise ratio is decreased if stray excitation light is detected by the emission detector.

An ideal laser is one that emits only a fixed wavelength of light, with minimal fluctuation in that output. However, some lasers suffer from thermal sensitivity and color shifts, which can vary the collection of signal. For example, the power output can be widely variable if the temperature of the laser fluctuates. The most common method for solving such problems is to control the temperature of the lasers by active monitoring, and to monitor the power output with active feedback to keep the output constant.

Another troublesome feature of some lasers is spectral shifting. For diode lasers, there is a slight increase in the wavelength of the laser output as the temperature increases. Once again, this effect can be reduced with careful temperature regulation of the laser itself.

For laser-based scanning systems, it is important to consider the diameter of the laser beam as it impinges on the microarray. This laser spot size should approximate the size of the sampling pixel. If the laser spot size is greater than the pixel size, one loses spatial resolution because the beam illuminates regions outside the pixel.

**Table 2.1** Commonly available lasers and the properties of the appropriate fluorophores that each laser can excite

| LASER WAVELENGTH (nm) | DYES | PEAK EXCITATION | PEAK EMISSION |
|---|---|---|---|
| 409 | Alexa 430 | 431 | 541 |
| 473 | Cy-2 | 489 | 506 |
| | 5-FAM | 492 | 518 |
| | Fluor-X | 494 | 520 |
| | Alexa 488 | 495 | 519 |
| | R-phycoerythrin | 480, 546, 565[a] | 578 |
| 532/543 | Cy-3 | 550 | 570 |
| | Alexa 532 | 531 | 554 |
| | Alexa 546 | 556 | 573 |
| | POPO-3 | 534 | 570 |
| | PO-PRO-3 | 539 | 567 |
| | R-phycoerythrin | 568 | 575 |
| 594 | Cy-3.5 | 581 | 596 |
| | Alexa 568 | 578 | 603 |
| | Alexa 594 | 590 | 617 |
| 635/633 | Cy-5 | 649 | 670 |
| | BODIPY 630/650-X | 625 | 640 |
| 670 | Cy 5.5 | 675 | 694 |
| 690 | Cy 7 | 743 | 767 |

[a] R-phycoerythrin has two excitation peaks and can be excited by two different wavelength lasers.

The loss of spatial resolution can reduce the SNR at that pixel by including signal and background from neighboring pixels. This effect is less significant if the laser spot size is smaller than the pixel size. For a conventional laser-based scanner that is scanning with 10-μm resolution, the ideal laser spot size is marginally smaller than 10 μm.

When scanning a microarray with a laser-based system, the amount of light that is delivered to a given area, and therefore the emitted signal, is determined by two parameters: the power of the laser and how long that laser is centered on a given region (dwell time). For laser scanning systems there is a tradeoff between these two parameters. For low-powered laser systems, it is necessary to increase the dwell time to ensure that enough light is delivered to the spot. This results in longer scan times. For higher powered lasers, a faster scan is possible, but it is important that the dwell time be short enough to prevent photobleaching. Photobleaching is easily measured by quantifying any decrease in image intensity when repetitively scanning the same microarray.

### Light Collection

Some of the most important issues to consider when evaluating light collection components include (for general review refer to Reichman, 1994 and Booth and Hill, 1998):

Lenses
Filters and mirrors
Optical design
Optical detectors

### LENSES

For a laser-based scanning system, the choice of lens for the system is not as critical as it is for a CCD-based system. This is mostly because of the functions of lenses in the two systems. In a laser-based scanning system, the lens is simply used to focus the light onto the sample and then collect emitted light back from the sample. A lens in a CCD-based imaging system not only serves the functions given earlier, but must also relay an image of the sample back to the detector. The following discussion of lenses relates primarily to CCD-based imaging systems.

In a CCD system there is always a tradeoff in maximizing the imaging area while minimizing optical aberrations. A common approach is to use relatively large diameter (and expensive) lenses. The problem with such lenses is the appearance of comet tails, also known as "flare." Such flaring greatly increases the noise of the image, thus reducing the SNR. One can also use smaller lenses with smaller imaging areas to collect smaller area images. These smaller images are then stitched together to create the full image. However, stitching images can introduce artifacts in the images caused by mechanical variations in signal repeatability among scans. In addition, a CCD collects light from the entire field of view simultaneously, so that signals from bright spots may mask signals from neighboring weak spots. Collecting light from the entire field of view can also increase the overall background.

Another lens consideration is image nonuniformity. Typically, only a limited area of the imaging field of a given lens is uniform. Toward the edge of the imaging field, there is a large increase in optical aberrations. Although this can be corrected through the use of additional lenses, such an approach is typically not used because optical efficiency is of paramount importance for microarray imaging. The introduction of additional lenses simply reduces optical throughput. Therefore the most common solution is to use only a portion of the imaging area and to collect more images.

Because of the desire to collect as large an image as possible, CCD systems typically have low-magnification lenses. Inherent in these lenses is a low efficiency of light collection, expressed as numerical aperture (NA). Since sensitivity is proportional to the square of the NA, a reduction in NA greatly attenuates the sensitivity of the system and reduces the SNR. For CCD systems, it is not uncommon to have an NA of about 0.3, whereas laser scanning systems may have an NA on the order of 0.6 to 0.7 or greater.

FILTERS AND MIRRORS

Fluorescence-based microarray imaging relies on the fact that one can illuminate a fluorophore with one wavelength of light, and that the fluorophore then emits light at a longer wavelength. This effect, known as the Stokes shift, is a fundamental property of fluorescence microscopy (see Rost, 1991). However, fluorophores are not tuned to a single wavelength, but instead absorb and emit across a range of wavelengths. A properly designed scanner must optimize the delivery and collection of only the appropriate wavelengths of light. This is achieved through single-wavelength lasers and careful selection of dichroic mirrors and emission filters.

A dichroic mirror is usually used to pass light of certain wavelengths and to reflect light of longer wavelengths. Dichroic mirrors are central to the epifluorescence microscopy design. The only caveat to heed when using dichroic mirrors is that they are not optically perfect. Regardless of the quality of the dichroic, there is *always* a small percentage of light that reflects when it is supposed to transmit and vice versa. Detection of stray photons that were not generated by the illuminated fluorophore degrades the SNR.

An alternative to using a dichroic mirror is to physically separate the excitation and emission light paths. This eliminates any problems associated with inadequacies of dichroic mirror coatings. Physically isolated optical paths are more difficult to engineer, may be more costly to produce, and do have the inherent limitation of reducing collected light (though not as much as a dichroic mirror). However, the endpoint of such detail is the sought-after increase in the SNR.

**Optical Design**

SIMULTANEOUS LASER-BASED SCANNING
The DNA that is hybridized on a microarray is stained with two fluorophores, most commonly Cy3 (green excitation light) and Cy5 (red excitation light). To create a microarray image, it is necessary to scan the microarray at both fluorescence excitation wavelengths. There are two different possible scanning approaches. A *sequential* scanner acquires one image at a time and then builds the ratio image after acquisition has been completed. A *simultaneous* scanner acquires both images at the same time.

What are some of the considerations when evaluating simultaneous vs. sequential scanners?

Advantages of a simultaneous scanner:

- Simultaneous scans are faster than a scanner requiring an independent scan from each channel.
- There is no need for image alignment after the scan is completed. Image alignment is often necessary when using a sequential scanning system to compensate for slight movements of the slide from one scan to the next and inherent mechanical variations in stage movements. A simultaneous scanner does not have these problems.
- If the software permits it, either of the raw data images [from each fluorophore (Cy3 or Cy5)] or the composite ratio image can be viewed while scanning. In addition you have full control of the display while scanning—capabilities such as zooming, brightness, and contrast control—and can perform real-time analysis.

The advantage of real-time image display is that problems with the slide or the scan can be identified before completing a whole scan (real-time scanning can also be done with sequential scanners, but only in one channel at a time). For example, if the slide is poorly spotted, or if the photomultiplier tube (PMT) settings are not optimal, this can be seen in the first few seconds of the scan and can save the trouble of wasting a complete scan.

Disadvantage of a simultaneous scanner:

- The most common concern with simultaneous scanning is the potential problem of crosstalk. With the appropriate optical design, crosstalk can be reduced.

What effect does simultaneous vs. sequential scanning have on the quality of the image? With an appropriate optical design, there may be no degradation in image quality that is due to crosstalk in a simultaneous scanner. With a sequential scanner, the images may not align perfectly, although this can be corrected with current software implementations.

## Optical Detectors

CHOICE OF OPTICAL DETECTOR

There are several choices in optical detectors, including photo-multiplier tubes, CCD cameras, and avalanche photodiodes (see Inoue and Spring, 1997, and Booth and Hill, 1998). Each of these components has both advantages and disadvantages, which are discussed below.

For a broadband illumination system, the most obvious detector is a CCD camera. Although the CCD camera allows the acquisition of a series of images that can be stitched together, there are significant performance considerations with such a detection system. CCDs have an inherent "read" noise. This noise refers to variability in the signal that arises from simply reading the values that are stored on the CCD sensor. This read noise can be in the range of 6–8 electrons (or a few counts on a 14-bit digitizer) compared with a virtually zero read noise from a PMT or an avalanche photodiode (although avalanche photodiodes suffer from significantly higher internal noise levels than either a CCD or PMT).

Detectors can introduce noise into the system and affect the SNR (see Booth and Hill, 1998). The *dark current*, for example, is measured in electrons per second and is introduced by the photomultiplier tubes or any photon-detecting device. This noise originates from thermal emissions from the photosensor, such as a photocathode, and/or leakage current through the dynodes of the PMT. In some cases electronic noise is included in the dark current values.

Dark current noise can be reduced to negligible levels through two approaches:

1. Selecting PMTs that show very low dark current levels.
2. Ensuring that the dwell time of the laser on each pixel is very short. This guarantees that the number of dark current electrons generated for each pixel is negligible.

Another important consideration is the quantum efficiency of the detector. CCDs typically have a much higher QE (in the range of 40%—although current backlit CCDs can have QE values as high as 85%). This QE is much higher than that of a PMT, which typically has a QE of about 15%. However, the backlit CCDs with higher QEs are much more difficult to produce with high quality, and hence are much more expensive.

One of the tradeoffs with a CCD sensor is a much more limited dynamic range than that with a PMT (Hamamatsu, 1994; Inoue and Spring, 1997). The most common way to increase the dynamic range of a CCD sensor is to increase the size of each sensing element (well). Unfortunately, this results in a reduction in spatial resolution, requiring a higher magnification objective and thus more image stitching to acquire the same image.

Finally, with CCD sensors one must consider the length of time it takes to acquire an acceptable image. Depending on the quality of the CCD camera, image acquisition times can vary significantly.

The bottom line when examining systems with different optical detectors is to objectively measure the image quality by computing the SNR. For some users, the speed of image acquisition is equally or nearly equally important.

PMT CONSTRUCTION
The choice of PMT for use in a microarray scanner is of critical importance. An extremely large number of PMTs are commercially available, and the goal is to find one that meets the appropriate specifications for a microarray scanner. One issue to consider is wavelength sensitivity. Not all PMTs detect light of different wavelengths with the same efficiency. For low-light microarray imaging, it is necessary to optimize the PMT selection to match the emission profiles of the most commonly used fluorophores. Failure to match the PMT wavelength with sample fluorescence can prevent optimization of the SNR.

In addition to variations in sensitivity, PMTs are also available in different physical shapes. There are end-on and side-on PMTs.

This terminology refers to the location of the photosensing region. End-on PMTs offer the advantage of a circular imaging area that is also more uniformly sensitive than the square side-on PMT imaging area. However, the choice of end-on PMTs is more limited when considering spectral sensitivity. In practice, one typically only uses a modest percentage of the effective photosensing area, and the area that is utilized is fixed. Therefore, nonuniform sensitivity is a small tradeoff to get a PMT with optimum spectral sensitivity.

LINEARITY OF THE PHOTOMULTIPLIER SYSTEM

When evaluating the linearity of the detection system in a PMT-based microarray scanner, there are two issues to consider, only one of which is significant: (1) Is the response linear over a wide range of incident light for a given PMT voltage (or gain setting)? (2) Is the response linear as the voltage (gain) of the PMT is changed?

It is important that the response over a wide range of incident light be linear for a fixed PMT setting (figure 2.3). This means that after the voltage of the PMT is set to some value, spots that vary significantly in intensity can be measured accurately.

It is much less important that the response be linear as the voltage of the PMT is changed. In fact, as the voltage of the PMT is changed, the response is highly nonlinear. In general, this is not an issue because one does not change the PMT voltage while scanning.

What does this mean for the user? For example, changing the voltage on the PMT from 200 to 400 V results in a different change in gain than when the voltage is changed from 400 to 600 V. Nevertheless, for a given voltage, the output of the PMT is linear over a wide range of emission signals. It is important to note that even if the PMT voltages for the red and green channels are different from each other, the gain is constant in both cases.

SIGNAL-TO-NOISE RATIO VS. PMT VOLTAGE (GAIN)

Without question, one of the most common misconceptions about microarray imaging is that a brighter image is a better image. The

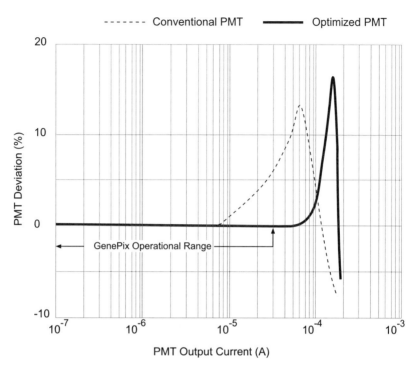

**Figure 2.3** For the GenePix microarray scanner from Axon Instruments, careful selection of optimized PMTs ensures linearity over a wide range of incident photons (PMT output current). (Adapted from Hamamatsu.)

easiest way to get a brighter image is simply to increase the gain of the PMTs. However, as mentioned earlier, the most important factor when evaluating image quality is the SNR.

Increasing the gain of the PMT does not necessarily increase the SNR. As the PMT gain is increased, there is an equivalent increase in the noise. The end result is that there is virtually no change in the SNR. While some argument can made that the PMT voltage has to be higher than a minimal value to detect anything at all, there is little point in pushing the PMT voltage to its extremes to get a brighter image (figure 2.4).

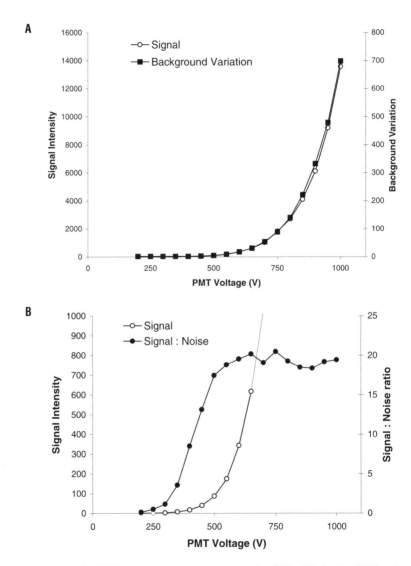

**Figure 2.4** Increasing the PMT voltage does not improve the SNR. (*A*) As the PMT voltage is increased, both the signal and the noise are scaled uniformly. (*B*) The SNR does not improve as the PMT voltage is increased. Note: On the right side the signal has been clipped to illustrate that only when the signal approaches the detection limits for this microarray does one see an appreciable effect on the SNR.

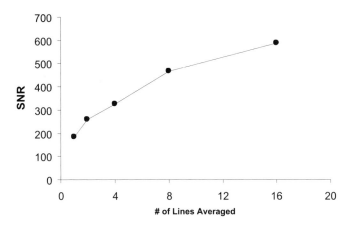

**Figure 2.5**  Line averaging increases SNR.

SIGNAL-TO-NOISE RATIO IN TERMS OF LINE AVERAGING OR
LINE INTEGRATION

In contrast to increasing the PMT gain, averaging (or integrating)
an image can increase the SNR. For the purposes of this discussion, line averaging is effectively the same as line integration. When
the same line is repetitively scanned, the total amount of signal
collected increases linearly as the number of lines being averaged
increases (in line-averaging mode, this signal is simply divided by
the number of lines averaged). However, in contrast to the signal,
the noise of the system only increases as the square root of the
number of lines averaged. As a result, as the number of lines averaged or integrated increases, the signal increases in a greater proportion than does the noise. The end result is a favorable increase
in the SNR (figure 2.5).

**Signal Collection and Processing**

The average user of a microarray scanner is aware that light is
being emitted from the microarray slide and that the scanner is
somehow converting this into a digital image on the computer
screen. This section outlines some of the signal processing that

must occur for the conversion of photons (reaching an optical detector) into a digital computer signal.

PMT SIGNAL PROCESSING

The output of a PMT operating in a conventional mode is not a digital signal but a continuous analog voltage that must be digitized. One must realize that since the laser beam is scanned continuously, a steady stream of photons are hitting the PMT during scanning. The scanner must determine which photons ultimately belong to each image pixel. There are two solutions for allocating photons to the correct pixel: integration and passive filtering.

Integration uses electrical integrators to continuously add incoming PMT signals to the current signal during each sample time, or pixel dwell time. After the sampling time is complete, the integrator is reset to 0 and the process recommences for the next pixel. In reality, integration is not so simple. The reset of an integrator is electrically very noisy. Scanning speeds are also so high that a simple integrator is not fast enough to ensure that the entire PMT signal is collected. One cannot afford simply to throw away photons when the electronics are reset or cannot keep up. As a result, a series of integrators that are tightly timed must be implemented to ensure maximum optical efficiency. This is a much more sophisticated and expensive solution, but it ensures maximum signal collection and maximum SNR.

An alternative method is to use passive filters. This approach typically uses a conventional resistor-capacitor (RC) circuit to accumulate the signal for one pixel. The signal must then passively discharge completely before the onset of the next pixel. There are several problems with passive filtering. When a very large signal hits this circuit, it takes much longer for the RC circuit to discharge. The net effect of this is that signal bleeds through into the next pixel or, under extreme conditions, the next several pixels. This manifests itself quite obviously in a microarray image as single-pixel-width "streaks" in the image. If the scanner is a bidirectional scanner (i.e., the laser scans from right to left and then

A

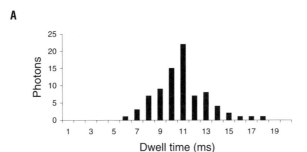

B

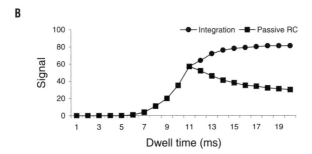

**Figure 2.6** Integration vs. passive acquisition of PMT signals. (*A*) The histogram shows the number of photons detected by a PMT in a 20-μsec dwell time. (*B*) The graph indicates the signal buildup and final value measured by the two types of systems. Note that while the signal in the passive RC circuit decays to a value less than the peak by the end of the sample time, the signal in the integrator circuit maintains its peak value until the end of the sample time.

from left to right on the next line), one can see streaks that alternate in direction. A second problem with the passive filter approach is that not all of the signal can be collected. Regardless of which approach is used, the end result is an analog signal that can be digitized for computer processing (figure 2.6).

ANALOG-TO-DIGITAL CONVERSION

The output of the PMT processing circuit is an analog signal that must be digitized. Digitization technology has been around for decades and is well established. For general reviews of electronics, see Diefenderfer, 1979, and Booth and Hill, 1998. When considering microarray imaging, there really are two digitization issues: (1) where the digitization is done and (2) the quality of the digitizer.

Most PMT-based scanners produce 16-bit images, which require 16-bit digitizers. Although there is a plethora of 16-bit digitizers on the market, it is imperative that one be chosen that shows extremely low digitization noise. Figure 2.7 shows two examples of 16-bit digitizers, both of very high quality. It is apparent that a digitizer with a higher noise would create an elevated level of background noise, thus reducing the SNR.

A second consideration for digitization is the location of the digitizer. We have found that there can be extreme additions of noise if the digitizing process is done *inside* the host computer, since additional noise is introduced by the electrically noisy environment. Furthermore, signal degradation can occur when the analog signal is transferred from the scanner to the computer for digitization. An ideal scanner has a high-quality 16-bit digitizer embedded within the scanner, thereby avoiding signal degradation and maximizing the SNR.

## Data Extraction and Analysis

Having dealt with the acquisition of microarray images, we can consider microarray analysis software as working in three stages: data extraction (spot finding), primary data analysis (individual spot analysis), and secondary data analysis (whole microarray analysis). For reviews, see Basarsky et al., 2000, and Zhou et al., 2000. We assess the role of the SNR at each stage.

## Data Extraction and SNR

Once a microarray has been scanned to produce an image, the user is faced with innumerable choices among methods of extracting the data. The fundamental aim of data extraction and analysis in

A

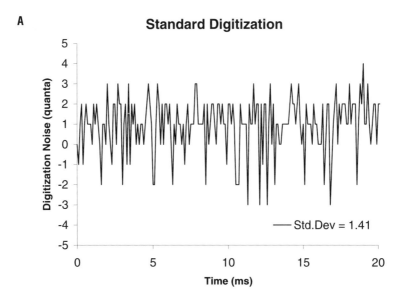

B

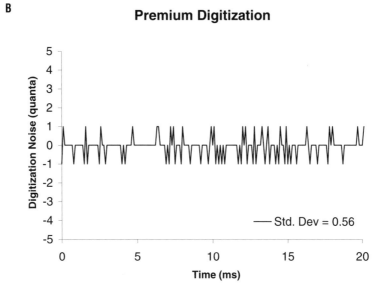

**Figure 2.7** The quality of the digitization process is affected by the quality of the analog-to-digital converter. The top panel (*A*) shows the noise apparent in an industry-standard digitizer, while the panel on the bottom (*B*) shows the noise from a premium digitizer.

any scientific field should always be data integrity. Microarray analysis software should separate the extraction of the raw data from its analysis; that is, one should never allow a quality measure, such as the SNR, to influence the extraction of raw data. In particular, one should not attempt to rectify deficiencies in slide preparation or scanner operation at the data extraction stage. Applied to the use of software to quantitate microarrays, a commitment to data integrity has a number of implications.

First, one must be careful to distinguish between data display and data analysis, and to keep the two separate. Although any number of image-filtering techniques can be used to improve the display of a microarray image, one should never alter the underlying pixel values that are analyzed. For example, median filtering of an image can improve the appearance of the image by modifying pixel values, but it should never modify the pixel values in the image that is analyzed. It is preferable not to filter the image in this way, but instead to calculate median intensity values for each feature on the microarray, which has the same effect as median filtering, but does not alter the raw data.

Second, when faced with an image analysis problem such as locating features of DNA and their local backgrounds, one should use a method that is independent of the particular quantities that are being measured. For example, one should not locate microarray features based on a maximization of signal-to-noise ratio, or a minimization of the local background. Some software packages allow the user to choose where to crop tails from background and feature pixel intensity distributions. Cropping the tails may make the data look better, but this may be a case of using a quality measure (SNR) to generate one's data, instead of extracting the data and then measuring its quality by calculating the SNR.

**Individual Spots and SNR**

Once one has the (presumably unadulterated) raw pixel values, one must decide how to identify an individual spot and its background in order to calculate its SNR. Independent of useability features such as speed and accuracy, two key qualities for any spot-finding algorithm should be robustness (it should succeed for many different images) and reproducibility (it should produce the same results when repeated).

Manual methods are very robust (i.e., one can usually find features by eye), but are not always reproducible (i.e., manually find the spots on the same image twice, and you will produce two different datasets). The variability increases when two individual users attempt to find the features manually. Automatic methods, with or without some manual intervention, are preferable, as long as the manual intervention does not compromise reproducibility.

The quest for automation and reproducibility has driven the development of proprietary "spot-finding" algorithms. Although these algorithms have existed for years for general image processing, new efforts have been made to optimize them for use with microarray images. They are discussed in detail in chapter 3 by Shah and Shams, and by Zhou and colleagues (2000).

Originally, microarray features were defined with simple circles and no attention was paid to the variability within the spot. As more sophisticated commercial packages have become available, the image processing and the finding of spots have become more quantitative. For example, many microarray image analysis packages support noncircular features (the noncircular feature is most likely an artifact of the printing process, but factors such as spot shape can affect the calculation of signal and background). Other packages take the quantitation to the next level, effectively filtering out selected pixels within the feature itself. Intraspot variability is also an artifact of printing and processing and can affect the quantitation of microarray data.

A local background method of analysis is preferable to a global background method because it takes into account the local variations in background levels across the microarray. The size of the local background region is, however, somewhat arbitrary. It must be large enough to provide a representative sample of background pixels, but not so large as to seriously compromise computational performance. One must exclude pixels from neighboring features, and one should also exclude pixels from the feature/background boundary because they cannot be placed reliably in either the feature or the background. A circular spot with a diameter of 100 μm contains about 80 feature pixels (using 10-μm pixels).

One method of determining local background is to draw a circular background region with a diameter three times that of the spot. Excluding pixels from neighboring features and the feature/ background boundary (e.g., an annulus around the spot with a 2-pixel width), such a local background region contains between 400 and 500 pixels, which is roughly five or six times the number of pixels in the spot. Such a method for determining local background can be implemented as a fully automated algorithm in software and satisfies the requirements of robustness and reproducibility (figure 2.8).

The next decision to make is how to calculate whole feature values for the feature and local background intensities from the pixel values. Typically, the choice is between the mean intensities and the median intensities. Median intensities are often preferred to mean intensities because they are not as seriously affected by extreme values at either end of a distribution.

The SNR for an individual feature can therefore be calculated using a local background technique:

(median feature intensity – median local background intensity)/ background standard deviation

How much does the consideration of internal spot variability, shape, size, etc. affect the final expression ratio? More work needs to be done in order to determine whether the extra efforts are worth it. Currently, there is no standard for analysis. This measure can be used as a quality control criterion for individual spots or one can use the data for whole microarray tests.

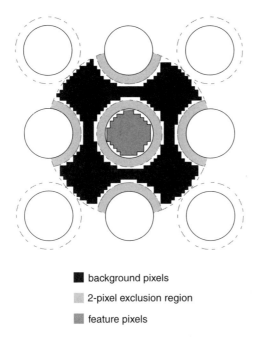

&#9632; background pixels

2-pixel exclusion region

&#9632; feature pixels

**Figure 2.8** Scheme to illustrate which pixels are included in the calculation of the feature signal and feature background, or excluded from all calculations.

### Whole Microarrays and SNR

Having the signal-to-noise data for each spot on a microarray enables one to calculate whole microarray quantities such as the mean or median SNR. These can be used as quality control criteria. Although an SNR of 3 is widely regarded as the minimum signal that can be reliably quantified, experience with many microarrays shows that a median SNR of 10 is readily achievable, often with median SNRs for whole microarrays of between 20 and 50. A microarray with an SNR of less than 10 may still be useful, but it points to some deficiency in slide preparation or scanner operation.

Using the median SNR for a whole microarray as a quality control criterion is most effective as part of a more extensive quality control effort. Other quality control criteria, such as the median background intensity, the median signal-to-background ratio, and the number of saturated pixels, provide additional indicators of data quality.

### Ratio Calculation and SNR

The next step in the process of analyzing and quantifying micro-array data involves calculating ratios. There are several different ways to calculate a ratio between two images, and the ratio calculations may affect SNR differently. In addition, it may be necessary to compare data between arrays and therefore a method of normalizing the data is needed.

Before all the ratios are calculated for every feature on an expression microarray, the two wavelength images must be "balanced." This can be done either with the hardware (by adjusting either the laser power or the detector gain) or in software (by simply multiplying an image with a balance factor). One can also normalize just the ratio calculations, after the data extraction.

What are the effects of applying a normalization factor to the data? Is it better to normalize with the hardware or the software? Empirically, the two methods should be the same. However, many software packages do not allow the multiplication of an image for balancing by a factor greater than 3, indicating that it might be best to normalize and balance in the hardware first. Normalization in software is strictly linear (one simply multiplies an image by a constant), whereas normalization and balancing using laser power and PMT gain for a scanner will not be linear. Normalizing with the hardware ensures that the balancing of the images does not extend beyond the dynamic range of the system. For example, one might multiply an image by a factor that causes features to exceed the 16-bit dynamic range of a TIFF file.

As we noted earlier, median intensities are often preferred to arithmetic mean intensities because they are not as seriously affected by extreme values at either end of a distribution. The *ratio of medians* is the ratio of the background-subtracted median pixel intensity at the second wavelength to the background-subtracted median pixel intensity at the first wavelength.

Mean intensities are familiar quantities, but they can be significantly skewed by extreme values at either end of a distribution. However, calculating the mean allows one to evaluate the variability of the data. This variability is reported as the standard deviation. The *ratio of means* is the ratio of the arithmetic mean of the background-subtracted raw pixel intensities at the second wavelength to the arithmetic mean of the background-subtracted raw pixel intensities at the first wavelength.

An alternative to computing the ratio from calculated means and medians of each whole feature is to compute the ratio on a pixel-by-pixel basis, and then to calculate the arithmetic mean and median of these many ratio values. An advantage of this approach is that a nonspecific signal, which appears in both wavelength images, has less of an effect than when the feature is treated as a whole. The *median of ratios* is the median of the pixel-by-pixel ratios of pixel intensities that have had the median background intensity subtracted. The *mean of ratios* is the arithmetic mean of the pixel-by-pixel ratios of the raw pixel intensities.

The regression ratio is another method of computing the ratio that does not require rigidly defining the background and foreground pixels. This is the most objective of the methods. All of the pixels within a circle that is larger than the diameter of the feature of interest are used. The relationship between wavelength 1 and wavelength 2 is determined by computing a linear regression between these two populations of pixels. The slope of the line of best fit (least-squares method) is the regression ratio. The coefficient of determination provides a measure of the level of accuracy of the fit. However, because the regression ratio does not make any assumptions about which pixels are feature pixels and which are background pixels, saturating pixels can skew the regression ratio because they heavily weight the slope of the best-fit line.

On a good array, all of the different ratio measurements tend to converge. If the regression ratio is significantly different from the other ratio quantities for some of the features, these features should be examined in more detail to determine the cause of the deviation.

Alternatively, microarray data can be normalized after the data are extracted from the image. In this case, assumptions are made about the distribution of ratio values across the array. In the most common form of normalization for an expression microarray, an assumption is made that the ratio distribution is normal and the mean should be near the value of 1 (Chen et al., 1997). This would be true in a case where most genes did not change their expression between two conditions. The shifting of a ratio distribution does not change the SNR, but assumptions must be accepted in order to interpret the data. An example of the use of this form of normalization is global normalization, such as that used by the Affymetrix system.

### Microarray Quality Control

How does one know whether a particular microarray should be included in an overall analysis? To date, very little quality control for the inclusion of microarray data has been described. It is likely that subjective, qualitative factors form acceptance criteria.

By carefully defining and quantifying particular features of a microarray image, acceptance criteria can be elevated to an objective, quantitative procedure. The signal-to-noise ratio can be used as a critical parameter for data acceptance. As discussed earlier, one can calculate the median or median SNR for all the features on an array. The acceptance threshold can then be set to a particular level, such as 10, and the array can be objectively judged to pass or fail that criterion. However, this approach is limited. The ultimate quality control would take into account a number of parameters such as spot size, raw intensities, and signal variation, as well as background variation, number of saturating pixels, and others. Reducing the multitude of parameters that can be extracted from a

**Table 2.2** Example of a portion of a quality control report generated in GenePix Pro microarray analysis software

| | VITAL STATISTICS | | | |
| --- | --- | --- | --- | --- |
| | *635 nm* | *532 nm* | *THRESHOLD* | *RESULT* |
| Median signal-to-background | 17.525 | 14.443 | >10 | Pass | Pass |
| Mean of median background | 167 | 142.305 | <200 | Pass | Pass |
| Median signal-to-noise | 19.308 | 16.817 | >10 | Pass | Pass |
| Features with saturated pixels | 0 | 0 | ≦3 | Pass | Pass |
| Not found features | 0/100 (0%). | | <7% | Pass |
| Bad features | 0/100 (0%). | | <7% | Pass |

Source: Axon Instruments, Inc.

microarray image to a single score would greatly assist in developing a standard procedure or test for the acceptance of microarray data (table 2.2).

## Conclusion

Each step in microarray creation, imaging, and analysis can affect the SNR of each feature on a microarray. The SNR can be optimized in every microarray experiment by careful preparation of the hybridized microarray sample itself. The glass-coating process must be designed to maximize uniformity and specific target binding, and to minimize all sources of background. All nucleic acid components must be carefully prepared, purified, and stored to ensure good hybridization efficiency and the highest possible signal levels.

The characteristics of the fluorescence imaging system also affect the SNR. The ultimate performance of any imaging system is the result of the contribution of all of its components—it cannot be determined by any one component or specification. However, different components affect the SNR in different ways. Sample excitation by a broad band of light delivers lower power, resulting in lower emission from the sample. In contrast, lasers deliver high-powered light at very specific wavelengths, for maximum light emission. Proper filtering keeps stray laser light out of the detector to minimize background signal. The dwell time and laser power must be optimized to maximize the signal and minimize photobleaching. Emitted light can be collected by a CCD array or a PMT.

A CCD collects light from a large area simultaneously. CCD images can have increased background owing to the large light collection area, and often require stitching to create a complete image. A CCD also has a lower dynamic range than commonly used PMTs, but an advantage of a CCD is that it is easy to change the dyes used by changing the filters.

In a fluorescent imaging system, PMTs must be chosen with response profiles that match the emission spectra of the dyes. The PMT response should be linear over a wide range of incident light for any given voltage, and it should be linear as the voltage changes. Increasing the PMT voltage may generate an image that appears brighter to the eye, but it also increases the noise, thereby reducing the SNR.

Averaging multiple scan lines decreases noise and can be used to improve detection limits and increase the confidence of each feature measurement. The process of converting the analog signal from the PMT into a digital signal (A-D conversion) can also contribute to noise. Using a low-noise digitizer and locating it outside the host computer can minimize noise.

Although the SNR is a powerful measure of quality for microarrays, features should be located based on raw data, not SNR maxima or local background minima. To increase confidence in feature measurements, spot-finding algorithms should be robust and reproducible with appropriate local background correction methods.

The signal-to-noise ratio is a powerful tool for assessing the quality of fluorescent microarray data. Minimizing variations in each component of the equation (i.e., signal, background, and background noise) increases the confidence in the results and allows more accurate interpretation of low-expressing genes. Taking these issues into consideration, the SNR can be used as quality measure for a whole microarray.

## References

Basarsky T, Verdnik D, Zhai J, and Wellis, D (2000). Overview of a microarray scanner: Design essentials for an integrated acquisition and analysis platform. In *Microarray Biochip Technology*, M. Schena, ed. Eaton Publishing, Natick, MA, pp. 265–284.

Booth KM and Hill SL (1998). *The Essence of Optoelectronics*. Prentice Hall, London.

Bowtell DDL (1999). Options available—from start to finish—for obtaining expression data by microarray. *Nature Genet (suppl)* 21: 25–32.

Brown PO and Botstein D (1999). Exploring the new world of the genome with DNA microarrays. *Nat Genet (suppl)* 21: 33–7.

Chen Y, Dougherty ER, and Bittner ML (1997). Ratio-based decisions and the quantitative analysis of cDNA microarray images. *J Biomed Optics* 2: 364–74.

Cheung VG, Morley M, Aguilar F, Massimi A, Kucherlapati R, and Childs G (1999). Making and reading microarrays. *Nat Genet (suppl)*, 21: 15–19.

Diefenderfer JA (1979). *Principles of Electronic Instrumentation, 2nd Ed.* Saunders College Publishing, Philadelphia.

Hamamatsu Photonics KK (1994). *Photomultiplier Tube. Principle to Application,* H. Kume, ed. Hamamatsu Photonics KK, Bridgewater, NJ.

Inoue S and Spring KR (1997). *Video Microscopy: The Fundamentals, 2nd Ed.* Plenum Press, New York.

Karpf AR, Peterson PW, Rawlins JT, Dalley BK, Yang Q, Albertsen H, and Jones DA (1999). Inhibition of DNA methyltransferase stimulates the expression of signal transducer and activator of transcription 1, 2, and 3 genes in colon tumor cells. *Proc Natl Acad Sci* 96: 14007–12.

Lander ES (1999). Array of hope. *Nat Genet (suppl)* 21: 3–4.

Pietu G, Alibert O, Guichard V, Lamy B, Bois F, Leroy E, Mariage-Samson R, Houlgatte R, Soularue P, and Auffray C (1996). Novel gene transcripts preferentially expressed in human muscles revealed by quantitative hybridization of a high density cDNA array. *Genome Res* 6: 492–503.

Reichman J (1994). *Chroma Handbook of Optical Filters for Fluorescence Microsopy*. Chroma Technology Corporation, Brattleboro, VT.

Rost FWD (1991). *Quantitative Fluorescence Microscopy*. Cambridge University Press, Cambridge, U.K.

Schena M, ed. (2000), *Microarray Biochip Technology*. Eaton Publishing, Natick, MA.

Schena M, ed. (1999). *DNA Microarrays. A Practical Approach*. Oxford University Press, New York.

Schena M and Davis RW (2000). Technology standards for microarray research. In *Microarray Biochip Technology,* M Schena, ed. Eaton Publishing, Natick, MA, pp. 1–18.

Song L, Varma CA, Verhoeven JW, and Tanke HJ (1996). Influence of the triplet excited state on the photobleaching kinetics of fluorescein in microscopy. *Biophys J* 70: 2959–68.

Zhou Y-X, Kalocsai P, Chen, J-Y, and Shams S (2000). Information processing issues and solutions associated with microarray technology. *Microarray Biochip Technology*, M. Schena, ed. Eaton Publishing, Natick, MA, pp. 167–200.

# 3 Microarray Image and Data Analysis

*Shishir Shah and Soheil Shams*

A microarray project involves acquisition and validation of large datasets containing different types of information and ranging from sequence data on the genes or clones placed on each slide to quantified expression values for each gene under different experimental conditions. Each project typically requires iterations of a series of processes. Figure 3.1 depicts the overall processing scheme, from experiment design and array fabrication, through array scanning, image analysis, and finally analysis of gene expression data. The analysis of expression data will likely lead to new hypotheses that will, in turn, require another iteration of experiment design, array fabrication and so on.

During each iteration, a process generates new data, which in turn can be used by other processes within the overall system. For example, data associated with the array fabrication process (containing information such as association of array configuration of gene IDs to spots, etc.) can be used by the image-processing system to automate many aspects of the process.

In the maturation of microarray technology, the informatics challenge is just developing. There are three major issues involved. The first is how to keep track of the information generated at the stages of chip production and hybridization experiment. The second is processing microarray images to obtain the quantified gene expression values from the arrays. The third is mining the information from the gene expression data. The goal of this chapter is to present these issues in detail and depict possible solutions.

In order to improve the overall life cycle of these experiments, accurate high-throughput analysis is a must. Since the final verification of a hypothesis is based on the outcome of data analysis, it

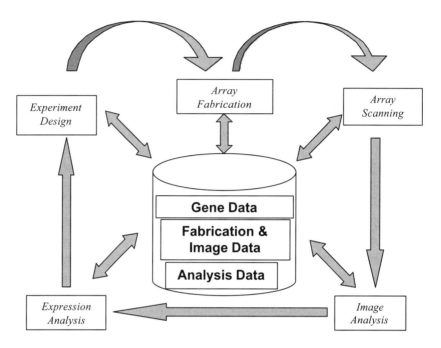

**Figure 3.1** The overall microarray information-processing system.

is imperative that the computations performed in the image analysis step be reliable and provide replicable, unbiased outputs. We discuss different image analysis techniques and compare their reliability through a set of controlled experiments.

In this chapter, first we present the informatics problems that emerge at the array fabrication stage. Then we describe the key issues involved in processing microarray images, along with the typical image characteristics. Problems involved in signal detection and spot localization are then addressed. Following this discussion, the next section illustrates a variety of ways to quantify the signal and to perform quality measurements for assessing the reliability of data and for revealing problems that occur during the array fabrication and hybridization processes. The different processing modes are compared and their effects on data reliability are presented at the end of the section. The final section briefly describes some of the issues and solutions for mining data and analyzing gene expression data.

### Array Fabrication Informatics

The array fabrication process may be conceptualized in four steps or subprocesses, each of which has its own set of data and/or parameters, as shown in figure 3.2. Array production begins with planning an experiment and selecting the genes or clones, also known as probes, to be printed on the arrays. In many cases these are selected from a preexisting database. Once a gene expression experiment has been planned, the first step is to design the layout of the microarray chips that will contain the probes of interest.

In each of the steps in figure 3.2, a large amount of information is produced and needs to be handled appropriately. The use of this information is not limited to the array fabrication process. Some of it may be useful in the subsequent processes, such as image processing and analysis of gene expression. The informatics challenge in array fabrication is to maintain a vast amount of information,

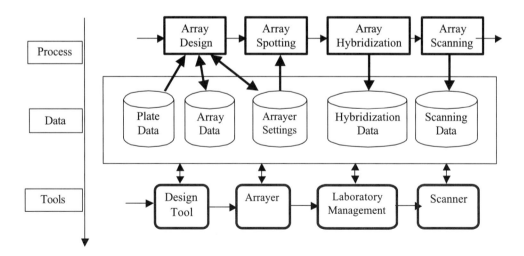

**Figure 3.2** The fabrication process.

organize it into a structured database for efficient access, and provide utilities for the design of microarray chips. These three issues are the central theme of this section.

### Information Management

It is essential to track the relevant data as it passes through the various stages of the microarray fabrication process. Each step in this process has its own set of data and/or parameters:

1. *Plate data.* Each plate may have a unique ID, an associated user name, and identifiers for each clone in each well.
2. *Array data.* Data related to an array may include layout information such as the spot density, the spacing between adjacent spots, and more important, information about the clones placed at each spot on the array.
3. *Configuration of arrayer and array spotting.* The arrayer configuration may include the number and type of pins, the number of pin cleansing cycles, etc. Some of these are parameters needed to set up the arrayer and some are those needed for tracking and logging purposes.
4. *Array hybridization conditions.* This may include the protocol and chemical buffers used and other experimental conditions.
5. *Array scanning conditions.* This includes the type of scanner and the parameters used when scanning an array. From a conventional point of view, array scanning is not included in the array fabrication process. However, from a laboratory information management point of view, it makes sense to keep data regarding *physical* operations on arrays in the same place for tracking purposes.

The major purpose of building the database system for array informatics is to facilitate access to information for designing the experiment, tracking problems and tuning the system, replicating chips and experiments, and sharing data with other processes. The key tasks can be categorized as follows:

1. *Experiment design.* The ability to browse through a plate database or obtain spot densities of existing arrays can provide useful information for decision making, such as the number of arrays to be produced or the number of duplicates needed for each clone.

2. *Problem tracking and system tuning.* Given a badly fabricated array or an erroneous data point, with an efficient database system the user can quickly trace back to the source of the problem and possibly remedy it through fine tuning of the array fabrication and experiment processes.

3. *Replicating arrays and experiments.* The user may want to replicate the same experiments on different arrays or vice versa. Having an efficient database system ensures that the information is available for precisely replicating the processing steps.

4. *Data sharing.* The information in the database is useful not only for array fabrication and experiments, but also for subsequent processes, such as image processing and analysis of gene expression. For example, image analysis software can take gene IDs as input and associate them with quantified values for each spot in the array.

The informatics problem in the array design cannot be solved by a database alone. It involves the implementation of the database infrastructure plus tools for navigation of the database, as well as software support for design of the array. The major components of this process are given below.

1. *Laboratory information management.* A necessary component is a management system that provides an access interface to the underlying array fabrication database. This is used to monitor the overall fabrication process by letting the user query different aspects of the fabrication process, update data step by step according to the progress of the experiment, and track the various operations performed on each spot in each array.

2. *Array design.* There should be an easy-to-use visual interface that enables the user to design or adjust the array layout based on the type of mechanical arrayer used and the design objectives. The system could also export the various arrayer parameter settings

or even generate complete programs to control the arrayer robot directly.

3. *Utilities for complex data manipulation.* The information flow in the fabrication process involves several transformations that cannot be handled using simple database operations. One example is the transformation of clone data from a set of plates (plate data) into spot data on the array (array data). Generation of the correct mapping is an essential component of array informatics since it relates the array data back to the plate data.

### Solutions to Data Management

There are many solutions to the data management problem. A simple and effective scheme can classify the data into categories according to different stages in the fabrication process. At the top level, there is a global structure that maintains the process information. In each category there is a skeleton table that links to the data in that category, and the top-level structure refers only to these skeleton tables. For each data category, a set of tables is provided, but the user is allowed to augment or replace them as desired. Software support is needed to provide simple navigation and management interfaces to the database. When browsing user-defined data, special interfaces are required to ask the user for the table information.

### Array Image Analysis

The fundamental goal of array image processing is to measure the intensity of the arrayed spots and quantify their expression values based on these intensities. In a more sophisticated and complete approach, the array image processing will also assess the reliability of the quantified spot data and generate warnings against possible problems during the array production and/or hybridization phases. Before these operations can be performed, the spots in the images must be identified. The specific properties of the spots are the central concern in the design of image-processing systems for micro-array images; in fact, the design of any effective image-processing system must be based on the specific properties of the images to be analyzed.

One of the primary concerns is the maximization of the signal-to-noise ratio in the raw image. One way to compute the SNR within an image is to compute the peak signal divided by the variation in the signal. If the scanning system generating the image has a poor SNR, an accurate quantification of individual spots becomes very difficult (see chapter 2). We characterize and model all imaging systems as linear, and hence noise characterization is implicit in the process. Knowledge of the functionalities of a particular imaging system can help in improving the SNR, thereby aiding in accurate analysis of the signal. Since the image is a function of the incident light or photons, a photomultiplier tube is used to detect the photons and quantize the value to report intensities in an image. Owing to thermal emissions and current leakage, electronic noise is introduced in the system. Such noise can typically be modeled as Gaussian-distributed white noise. One can reduce the amount of this noise in the image by controlling exposure time and gain while scanning.

The second noise type introduced in the system is proportional to the square root of incident photons (signal). Owing to the natural distribution of photons, as the number of incident photons is increased, the variability in this number also increases. Thus, as the intensity increases, the noise also increases.

The third and often significant source of noise is the substrate of the array slide. The substrate material used can contribute to background fluorescence, which reduces the sensitivity of the signal. Improper treatment of the slide surface will result in poor attachment of the DNA and hence will also reduce the resultant signal.

Finally, residual material and improper handling and drying of the slide will result in background fluorescence. The rest of this section highlights the requirements for reliable automated image analysis.

### Properties and Problems of Microarray Images

Most cDNA microarray images violate the following "ideal" properties:

1. All the subgrids should be the same size.
2. The spacing between the subgrids should be regular.
3. The distance between adjacent rows and columns should be the same.
4. The spots should be centered on the intersections of the lines of the rows and columns (the canonical position).
5. The size and shape of the spots should be perfectly circular and the same for all the spots.
6. The location of the grids should be fixed in images for a given type of slide.
7. No dust or other contamination should be on the slide.
8. There should be minimal noise in the images, thus a high signal-to-noise ratio.
9. There should be minimal and uniform background intensity across the image.

These violations of the ideal may be summarized as four issues: variation in spot position, irregular spot shapes and sizes, noise and contamination, and global problems that affect multiple spots.

Variation in spot position is caused by the mechanical limitations in the spotting process. Researchers are motivated to put as many spots as possible onto a single array to increase the efficiency of the hybridization experiments. The fundamental concern in the fabrication of the array is to make sure that the spots are not overlapping each other. Spots that are perfectly linearly aligned are a secondary concern.

Several sources contribute to the nonuniform positioning of the spots in the array. The pins may vibrate during the spotting, causing offsets. The spatial mapping between slides and scanned images may not be perfectly linear, causing the spacing between the adjacent columns to vary. Some of the spots may be "missing" from the grid owing to a lower-than-measurable expression level or empty wells in the plates used for array fabrication. The arraying apparatus might have vibrations caused by the mechanical motion of the robot.

Because the spot sizes are on the scale of 100–300 μm, "fixing" the location of the grids on each image means that the spots must be placed with at least 10 μm precision (property 6). This requirement is prohibitively expensive to satisfy. Again, because the spots in a grid are typically printed with multiple pins, for the spots from each pin to align accurately, the group of pins has to be aligned to 10 μm accuracy as well (properties 1–4), which is another prohibitively expensive requirement. The existence of these positional variations in microarray images demands an intelligent spot localization operation, which must be carried out either by means of human eyes or by computer vision algorithms.

In addition to variation in position, the shape and size of the spots may fluctuate significantly across the array. The sizes of the droplets of DNA solution may vary, which will cause the size of the spots to change. Concentrations of the DNA and salt in solution may also change with time, making the shape of spots deviate from a typical circle and making the density of DNA vary within a spot. The contact space between the tips of the pins and the slide surface may change. The surface properties of the slides may vary from place to place. All these factors change the shape and size of the spots from what is expected. To obtain an accurate measurement of the hybridization strength, signal pixels need to be identified intelligently to take account of these problems.

Contamination is also a major source of problems in microarray image processing. From the procedure of spotting to hybridization experiments, dust floating in the air may land on the slides, often causing bright noise signals in the scanned images. Certain drying rates may cause little "bumps" in the spot surface, producing specular reflections in the images. Contamination may also come from splashes and drips of DNA solution from pins or impurities in the slide surface. Figure 3.3 (see also plate 2) shows examples of contamination in the image. One may see the small contamination

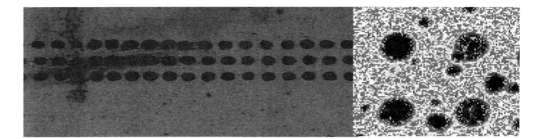

**Figure 3.3** Contamination in microarray images may be seen in both the background and inside the spots. See plate 2 for color version.

spots distributed in the background and the small contamination particles inside the spots with extreme intensity level. The best solution to these problems is to identify the contamination and remove it before making measurements.

There are also other factors that affect the quality of data in a larger area of the slides, such as glass quality, nonuniform temperature across the slide, scrapes by the pin when spotting, or bubbles during hybridization. All these global quality problems, as well as the local problems illustrated here, need to be handled either by human inspection or by image-processing systems. We briefly review some basic processing that can be performed to minimize noise in the images.

**Noise Suppression**

Imaging is modeled as a linear system where the image is obtained as an output of the ideal signal convolved with the impulse response of the imaging system. Noise suppression or filtering can be achieved by knowing the impulse response of the system and deconvolving the obtained image with it. Owing to the complexity of the imaging process and the other factors degrading the quality of the image, modeling this system as a linear system and hoping to find a perfect impulse response to that system is a rather simplistic view. In practice, one has to choose a filter based on an assumption of the noise process in the system. Filters can be broadly separated into two categories: linear and nonlinear (Duda and Hart, 1973; Haralick, 1979). The former are amenable to analysis in the Fourier domain and the latter are not.

Linear filters are good for removing Gaussian noise. Gaussian noise contains variations in intensity that are drawn from a normal distribution and is a good model for many kinds of sensor noise, including camera electronics. Any linear filter is implemented as a weighted sum of pixels in successive windows. Typically, the same pattern of weights is used in each window; thus the filter is spatially invariant and can be implemented using a convolution mask. Broadly speaking, any filter that is not a weighted sum of pixels is a nonlinear filter. Nonlinear filters can be spatially invariant if the same operation is performed regardless of the position in the image.

One of the simplest linear filters is implemented by local averaging, where the value of each pixel is replaced by the average of all the values in the local neighborhood. This is known as an average filter or a mean filter. If the weighting function is derived by the convolution of two uniform filters, it results in a triangular function, which gives more weight to closer neighborhood support. This is known as a triangular filter. More common is the Gaussian filter, which uses a Gaussian kernel. It is rotationally symmetric; thus the filtering performed is the same in all directions. Linear filtering removes high-frequency components, and the sharp details in images are lost. Distinct boundaries between spots and background will be replaced with gradual changes, and the ability to accurately locate a change will be sacrificed. One can implement smarter procedures in which the filter weights are adjusted so that more smoothing is done in relatively uniform areas of an image, which will typically be background regions.

In microarray images, we would like to quantify and analyze the raw data and understand the expression based on the differences in signal and background values. The use of linear filters may compromise the localization accuracy of the spots; thus they do not form an ideal choice even if the SNR improvement is shown to be significant.

An alternative approach is to use a median filter, in which each pixel value is replaced with the median of the intensities in the local neighborhood. This is an effective nonlinear filter that removes impulse and salt-and-pepper noise while retaining details. It is also effective in removing Gaussian noise to a large extent.

A useful variation on the theme of the median filter is the percentile filter, in which the center pixel in the window is replaced, not by the 50% (median) brightness value, but rather by the $p\%$ brightness value where $p\%$ ranges from 0% (the minimum filter) to 100% (the maximum filter).

In an effort to preserve details within the image while reducing the noise, edge-preserving filters also form a good choice. The Kuwahara filter replaces the pixel value with the mean value of the local neighborhood region that has the smallest variance. This aids in preserving the mean signal and background values while removing impulse noise.

Improved filtering and noise suppression can be obtained by combining multiple filters and adaptively computing the weights for nonlinear filtering based on local statistics of the image (Shah and Aggarwal, 1997a). The nonlinear function used can be defined in terms of polynomials, neural networks, or other function-approximate schemes. To justify this approach, one must assume that the processes generating the image, blurring, and noise are all *stationary*—in the random process sense that the probability of a particular behavior does not depend on the image coordinates. This kind of stationarity is called "strict sense stationarity." This assumption holds true in most cases of microarray images. However, even images that violate this assumption will do so only mildly on the scale of interest, namely, small local windows. Optimizing the filter coefficients for an example microarray image results in improved noise removal over median filtering (figure 3.4 and plate 3).

**A.**  **B.**  **C.**

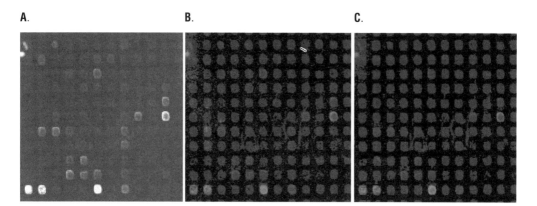

**Figure 3.4**  Comparison between median filtering (*B*) and combined local statistics adaptive filtering (*C*) as applied to an example microarray image (*A*). See plate 3 for color version.

## Spot Localization

The first step after suppression of noise is to localize the position and size of each spot in the face of the realities of spot position variation. The second step is to address shape irregularity and contamination problems through a signal pixel identification process. The last step is to deal with the global problems of spatial irregularities. The first two steps are discussed in this section. The process in the third step requires global quality information and will be discussed in the following section.

### Spot-Finding Methods for Resolving Spot Localization Errors

The goal of spot finding is to locate the signal spots in images and estimate the size of each spot. There are three different levels of sophistication in the algorithms for spot finding and they correspond to the degree of human intervention in the process. These are described here in order from most to least (in terms of the amount of manual intervention).

MANUAL SPOT FINDING

This method is essentially a computer-aided image-processing approach. The computer itself does not have any visual capabilities to "see" the spots, but provides tools to allow the users to tell the computer where each of the signal spots is in the image. Typically, a grid frame is manually placed on the image and manipulated to fit to the spots in the image. Because the spots may not be evenly spaced, the user may need to adjust the grid lines individually to align them with the arrayed spots. The user may also have to adjust some grid points to land onto the spots in the image. The size of each circle may also need manual adjustment to fit to the size of each spot. To conduct an accurate measurement, this method is prohibitively time-consuming and labor intensive for images that have thousands of spots. Thus considerable inaccuracy of the data may be introduced by human errors, particularly with arrays having irregular spacing between the spots and large variation in spot sizes.

SEMIAUTOMATIC SPOT FINDING

This approach usually uses algorithms to automatically adjust the location of the grid lines or individual grid points after the user has specified the approximate location of the grid. For example, the user may need to put down a grid and adjust its size to fit or indicate the location of the corners of the subgrids in the images. Then the spot-finding algorithm adjusts the location of the grid lines, or grid points, to locate the arrayed spots in the image. User interface tools are usually provided by the software to allow for manual adjustment of the grid points if the automatic spot-finding method has not correctly identified each spot.

This approach saves time over the manual spot-finding method since the user only needs to identify a few points in the image and make minor adjustments. The key issue for spot-finding algorithms here is to correctly identify the spots even at very low levels of intensity. In addition, the algorithm must deal effectively with two opposing criteria: (1) owing to variation in spot position, as described earlier, the algorithm must tolerate a certain degree of irregularity in the spot spacing and (2) the algorithm must not be distracted by contaminants that could be adjacent to a true arrayed spot.

AUTOMATIC SPOT FINDING

The ultimate goal of array image processing is to build an automatic system that utilizes advanced computer vision algorithms to find the spots without any human intervention. This method would minimize the potential for human error and would offer a great deal of consistency in data quality. Such a processing system would require the user to specify the expected configuration of the array (e.g., number of rows and columns of spots) and would automatically search the image for the grid position. Having found the approximate grid position, which specifies the centers of each spot, the system would examine the neighborhood to detect signal and background. Knowledge about the image characteristics would be incorporated to account for variabilities in microarray images, and the spot location, size, and shape would be adjusted to accommodate for noise, contamination, and uneven distribution.

**Spatial Segmentation of Signal and Background Pixels**

After the spot location is determined in the image, a small patch around that location (target region) can be used to quantify the spot expression level. The next step is to determine which pixels in the target region are due to the actual spot signal and which are due to background. In computer vision terminology, this operation is called "signal or image segmentation" (Pal and Pal, 1993). At this stage, the size and shape irregularities of the spots, and any contamination problem in the images, are the major concern in the algorithm design. A number of methods have been developed with different levels of sophistication. Their advantages and disadvantages are described in the following section.

PURE SPACE-BASED SIGNAL SEGMENTATION
Methods in this class use purely spatial information from the result
of spot finding to segment out signal pixels. After the spot finding
operation has been completed, the location and size of the spot is
determined. A circular mask of the computed size is placed in the
image at the determined position to separate the signal from the
background. It is assumed that the pixels inside the circle are due
to the true signal and those outside are background. The measurements are then performed on these classified pixels. These types of
methods are optimal when the spot-finding operation is effective
(i.e., spots have been correctly located and sized, the spot shapes
are close to perfect circles, and no contamination is present) (Price,
1984). Knowing the configuration of the array and the spacing between spots, the user can specify the number of pixels around the
spot that can be used to compute the background value.

However, irregularities of spot shape and size, as well as spot
contamination, are common and compromise the accuracy of space-
based measurements. In addition, spot contamination is still a large
issue in many microarray images. In the example shown in figure
3.5, nearly a 50% difference is observed between mean measurements made before and after the removal of contamination from
the image.

Two broad classes of spot shapes will cause problems with
pure space-based signal segmentation. First, "donut-shaped" spots,
which are often seen with many arraying systems, contain many
nonhybridized pixels within the circular spot area. Using this segmentation approach, these pixels will be mistakenly classified as
signal pixels. Second, noncircular spots (e.g., more elliptical spots)
cannot be fit perfectly with a round circle, thus causing some signal pixels to be considered as background and some background
pixels to be considered as signal.

This method of quantification is used by some available microarray image analysis software tools and is appropriate for a "quick
and dirty" look at most image data. However, it is not sufficiently
sophisticated to ensure accuracy of the quantified data in most
cases.

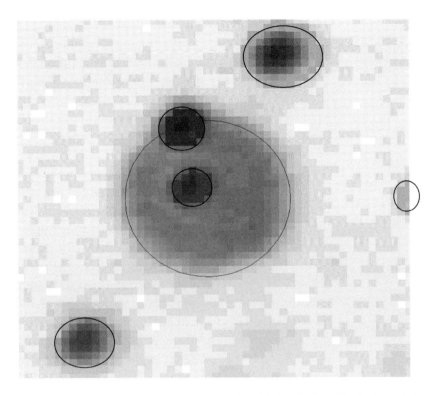

**Figure 3.5** Signal identification from spot-finding operation. All the pixels inside the blue circle in the center are considered as signal and the pixels outside as background according to this method. However, when contaminations exist, as outlined by small circles, measurement errors are introduced both in the signal and in the background regions. In this image, the mean signal intensity using purely spatial segmentation is 1232.8. After the contamination pixels are removed, the signal mean is 833.9; the difference is 48%. The mean background values are 112.7 and 27.6, respectively, before and after removal of the contamination: a difference of 300%.

PURE INTENSITY-BASED SIGNAL SEGMENTATION

Methods of this class use intensity information exclusively to segment out signal pixels from the background. They assume that the signal pixels are statistically brighter than the background pixels. As an example, suppose that the target region around the spot taken from the image consists of $40 \times 40$ pixels. The spot is about 20 pixels in diameter. Thus, from the total of 1600 $(40 \times 40)$ pixels in the region, about 314 $(\pi \times 10^2)$ pixels, or 20%, are signal pixels and are expected to have intensity values higher than those of the background pixels. To identify these signal pixels, all the pixels from the target region are ordered in a one-dimensional array from the lowest intensity pixel to the highest one, $\{p_1, p_2, p_3, \ldots, p_{2500}\}$, in which $p_i$ is the intensity value of the pixel of the $i$th lowest intensity among all the pixels. If there is no contamination in the target region, the top 20% pixels in the intensity rank may be classified as the signal pixels.

The advantage of this method is its simplicity and speed. The method works well when spot intensities are much higher than the background pixels. However, the method has disadvantages when dealing with spots of low intensities, negative expressions, or noisy images. When the signal intensity is low, the intensity distribution of the signal largely overlaps with that of the background. The signal and background pixels are not separable based on their intensity values alone. Applying this method will produce biased estimates of signal and background intensity values.

The shortcoming of a purely intensity-based segmentation method can be remedied by exploiting the spatial information. One simple method of obtaining spatial information is to segregate the target region into a potential signal region and a potential background region before conducting intensity-based segmentation. A circle can be placed in the target region based on the result of the spot finding. Pixels inside the circle are temporarily classified as signals and those outside as background pixels. The statistical differences in the two regions can be assessed and compared for signal segmentation. Two such methods, namely the Mann–Whitney test (Duda and Hart, 1973; Johnson and Wichern, 1998) and the trimmed measurement method are described next.

MANN–WHITNEY SEGMENTATION

Based on the result of the spot-finding operation, a circle is placed in the target region to include the spatial region of the spot. Because the pixels outside of the circle are assumed to be the background, the statistical properties of these background pixels can be used to determine which pixels inside the circle are signal pixels. The Mann–Whitney test is used to obtain a threshold intensity level (Chen et al., 1997). Pixels inside the circle having a higher intensity than the threshold intensity are identified as signal. This method works very well when the spot location is found correctly and there is no contamination in the image.

However, when contamination pixels exist inside the circle, they will be determined as signal pixels. This is because typical contamination will be seen as specular reflection and has an intensity higher than the background. If there are contamination pixels outside of the circle, or the spot location is not found correctly, so that some of the signal pixels are outside of the circle, these high-intensity pixels will raise the intensity threshold level. Consequently, the signal pixels with an intensity lower than the threshold will be misclassified as background. Applying the Mann–Whitney test to the example in figure 3.5, using an alpha value = 0.0001, the mean intensities quantified are 1235.7 for signal pixels and 32.5 for background pixels, respectively, producing about 50% and 20% deviation from the true values.

This method is also limited when dealing with weak signal and noisy images. When the intensity distribution functions of the signal and background are largely overlapping, classification of pixels based on an intensity threshold is prone to classification errors, resulting in measurement biases similar to but less severe than those observed in the pure intensity-based segmentation method.

TRIMMED MEASUREMENTS

This approach also combines both spatial and intensity information in segmenting the signal pixels from the background. In this method, a target circle is placed in the target region after the spot is located, where *most* of the pixels inside the circle are signal pixels, and *most* of the background pixels are outside of the circle. Owing to the shape irregularity, some signal pixels may leak out of the circle and some background pixels may get into the circle. These pixels may be considered as outliers in the sampling of the signal and background pixels. Similarly, contamination pixels may also be considered as outliers in the intensity domain. These outliers will severely change the measurement of the mean and total signal intensity. To remove the effect of outliers on these measurements, a fixed percentage of pixels from the intensity distribution of the pixels for both signal and background regions is trimmed off.

For example, a certain percentage of pixels at the high end of the intensity distribution, say 10%, is trimmed off from the pixels inside the circle. A certain percentage of pixels at the low end of the intensity distribution, say 20%, is also trimmed off from the pixels inside the circle, owing to their high possibility of being background. Whatever pixels remain inside the circle are considered signal pixels. The exact amount to be trimmed depends on the effectiveness of the spot-finding process and the quality of the image. A good estimate for these thresholds can be determined empirically. As long as the image quality does not change significantly (e.g., there is no major increase in contamination), these values can be used effectively. The major advantage of the trimmed measurement method is the robustness of the measurement against outliers, although this advantage is obtained at the expense of accuracy. When there are no outliers, trimming will reduce the measurement accuracy by reducing the number of pixels used in the calculation of the signal values. However, if there are significant pixels per spot and only a small percentage of the pixels is removed, this method can yield very good quantified values. Furthermore, by averaging the measurements from multiply replicated spots, this method should achieve very good performance.

Figure 3.6 illustrates the application of this method to the image in figure 3.5. The measurements derived from this method deviate about 30% from the true value, which is less of a deviation than from the other method discussed earlier. The major limitation of this method is the loss of shape information for the signal region after the trimming. However, the shape information is mostly important if it is used as part of the quality measurement associated with a spot and its considerable computational needs would re-

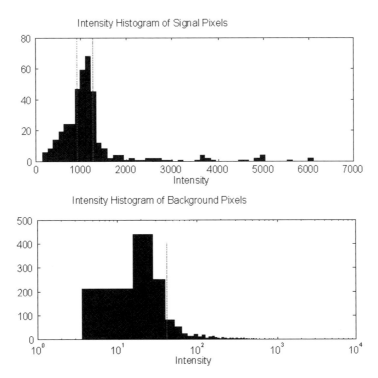

**Figure 3.6** Trimmed measurement method for identifying signal pixels. The upper figure plots the intensity histogram of the pixels inside the target circle. Thirty percent of pixels are trimmed off at the low-intensity side (left of the left vertical line). Twenty percent of pixels are trimmed from the high-intensity side (right of the right vertical line). The lower figure plots the histogram of the pixels outside the target circle. Thirty percent of the pixels are trimmed off at the high-intensity side of the histogram (right of the vertical dash line). The abscissa is in log scale to show the detail on the low-intensity side. The mean intensities are 1103 for signal and 19.6 for background. They differ from the true value by 32 and −29%.

quire a fully automated system for practical use. In semiautomatic systems, computational speed is of great concern. The trimmed measurement method provides the optimal choice of speed and accuracy.

INTEGRATING SPATIAL AND INTENSITY INFORMATION FOR
SIGNAL SEGMENTATION

The two methods discussed above use minimal amounts of spatial information, that is, the target circle obtained from spot localization is not used to improve the detection of signal pixels. Their design priority is to take measurements of spot intensity with minimal computation. These methods are useful in semiautomatic image processing because speed has strong priority and the user can visually inspect the quality of the data.

In a fully automated image-processing system, the accuracy of the signal pixel classification becomes a central concern. Not only does the correct segmentation of signal pixels offer accurate measurement of the signal intensity, but it also permits multiple quality measurements based on the geometric properties of the spots. These quality measures can be used to draw the attention of a human inspector to spots having values of questionable quality after the completion of an automated analysis. The correct classification of the signal pixels can be obtained by algorithms that use information from both spatial and intensity domains (Beulieu and Goldberg, 1989; Shah and Aggarwal, 1998, 1997b; Spann and Nieminen, 1988).

## Data Quantification and Quality Measurement

In gene expression studies, one is typically interested in the difference in expression levels between the test and reference mRNA populations. This translates into differences in the function of intensities on the two images. Under idealized conditions, the total fluorescent intensity from a spot is proportional to its expression. These idealized conditions are:

1. The preparation of the probe cDNA (through reverse transcription of the extracted mRNA) solution is done appropriately, so that the probe cDNA concentration in the solution is proportional to that in the tissue.

2. The hybridization experiment is done appropriately, so that the amount of cDNA binding on the spots is proportional to the probe cDNA concentration in the solution.

3. The amount of cDNA deposited on each spot during the chip fabrication is constant.

4. There is no contamination on the spots.

5. The signal pixels are correctly identified by image analysis.

In the following discussion, we assume that conditions (1) and (2) are satisfied. Whether these two conditions are truly satisfied should be controlled through the design of the experiments. For a measurement based on image analysis algorithms, we are mainly concerned about conditions (3)–(5).

**Quantification Methods**

In most cases, conditions (3)–(5) are violated. The DNA concentrations in the spotting procedure may vary from time to time and from spot to spot. Higher concentrations may result in larger spot sizes. When the contamination is on the spot, the signal intensity covered by the contaminated region is not measurable. The image processing may not correctly identify all the signal pixels; thus the quantification methods should be designed to address these problems. The common values computed are total, mean, median, mode, volume, intensity ratio, and the correlation ratio across two channels. The underlying principle for judging the best method is based on how well each of these measurements correlates to the amount of the DNA probe present at each spot location.

1. *Total.* The total signal intensity is the sum of the intensity values of all the pixels in the signal region. As indicated earlier, total intensity is sensitive to the variation in the amount of DNA deposited

on the spot, the existence of contamination, and the anomalies in the image-processing operation. Because these problems occur frequently, the total intensity may not be an accurate measurement.

2. *Mean.* The mean signal intensity is the average intensity of the signal pixels. This method has certain advantages over the total. Very often the spot size correlates to the DNA concentration in the wells during the spotting processing. Measuring the mean will reduce the error caused by the variation in the amount of DNA deposited on the spot. With advanced image processing that allows accurate segmentation of contamination pixels from the signal pixels, the mean should be the best measurement method.

3. *Median.* The median of the signal intensity is the intensity value that splits the distribution of the signal pixels into halves. The number of pixels above the median intensity is the same as those below. Thus, this value is a landmark in the intensity distribution profile. The advantage of choosing this landmark as the measurement is due to its resistance to outliers. As discussed in the previous section, contamination and problems in the image-processing operation introduce outliers in the sample of identified signal pixels. The mean measurement is very vulnerable to these outliers. When the distribution profile is unimodal, the median intensity value is very stable and it is close to the mean. In fact, if the distribution is symmetric in both high and lower intensity sides, the median is equal to the mean. Thus, if the image-processing operation is not sophisticated enough to ensure the correct identification of signal, background, and contamination pixels, the median is a better choice than the mean. An alternative to the median measurement is to use the trimmed mean, as discussed earlier. The trimmed mean is estimated after a certain percentage of pixels have been trimmed from the tails of the intensity distribution.

4. *Mode.* The mode of the signal intensity is the most likely intensity value and can be measured as the intensity level corresponding to the peak of the intensity histogram. It is also a landmark in the intensity distribution. Thus, it enjoys the same robustness against outliers offered by the median. The tradeoff is that the

mode becomes a biased estimate when the distribution is multimodal. This is because the mode value will be equal to one of the modals in the distribution, depending on which one is the highest. When the distribution is unimodal and symmetric, mean, median, and mode measurements are equal. Often the difference between mode and median values can be used as an indicator of the degree to which a distribution is multimodal.

5. *Volume.* The volume of signal intensity is the sum of the signal intensity above the background intensity. It may be computed as (the mean of the signal – mean of the background) × area of the signal. This method adopts the argument that the measured signal intensity has an additive component that is due to nonspecific binding, and this component is the same as that from the background. This argument may not be valid because the nonspecific binding in the background is different from that in the spot. Perhaps a better way is to use blank spots for measuring the strength of nonspecific binding inside spots. It has been shown that the intensity on the spots may be smaller than it is on the background, indicating that the nature of nonspecific binding is different between what is on the background and what is inside the spots. To a larger extent, the background intensity should be used for quality control rather than for signal measurement.

6. *Intensity ratio.* If the hybridization experiments are done in two channels, then the intensity ratio between the channels might be the only quantified value of interest. This value will be insensitive to variations in the exact amount of DNA spotted since the ratio between the two channels is being measured. This ratio can be obtained from the mean, median, or mode of the intensity measurement for each channel.

7. *Correlation ratio.* Another way of computing the intensity ratio is to perform correlation analysis across the corresponding pixels in two channels of the same slide. This computes the ratio between the pixels in two channels by fitting a straight line through a scatter plot of intensities of individual pixels. This line must pass through the origin, and its slope is the intensity ratio between the two

channels. This is also known as the regression ratio. This method may be effective when signal intensity is much higher than the background intensity. The motivation behind using this method is to bypass the signal pixel identification process. However, for spots of moderate to low intensities, the background pixels may severely bias the ratio estimate of the signal toward the ratio of the background intensity. Then the advantage of applying this method becomes unclear and the procedure suffers the same complications encountered in the signal pixel identification methods discussed earlier. Thus its advantage over the intensity ratio method may not be real. One remedy to this problem is to identify the signal pixels first before performing correlation analysis. Alternatively, one could identify the pixels that deviate within a specified amount from the mean of the intensity population.

Table 3.1 lists the results of mean, median, mode, and total quantification measurements using three signal pixel identification methods as applied to the image in figure 3.5. In the case of the trimmed method, 30% of the signal pixels were trimmed from the low-intensity side of the distribution and 20% from the high-intensity side. For background pixel identification, pixels in a three-pixel-wide ring outside the signal circle were discarded because of their potential for containing signal pixels "bleeding" into this region. In addition, 30% of the remaining background pixels were trimmed from the high-intensity side. The measurements were

**Table 3.1** Measurements using different quantification and image-processing methods

|              | MEAN    | MEDIAN  | MODE    | TOTAL   |
| ------------ | ------- | ------- | ------- | ------- |
| Combined     | 833.95  | 934.61  | 997.78  | 384,450 |
| Trimmed      | 1103.06 | 1109.42 | 1109.42 | 207,375 |
| Pure spatial | 1232.80 | 1076.05 | 1063.25 | 464,765 |

done after trimming. The combined intensity and spatial segmentation method was used to identify signal, background, and contaminated pixels before computing the intensity measurement. The measurements were based on the segregated regions.

Because of contamination in the image, the mean method from the combined segmentation is optimal. The median and mode measurements deviate about 10–15% from the mean. According to the trimmed method, the three measurements are very similar; they deviate about 30% from the mean of the combined technique. Without trimming, the mean measurement produces a 50% deviation; however, the median and mode estimates are essentially unchanged. Based on our experience and observations, the mean is the best measurement when using the combined and trimmed segmentation techniques. Without trimming, the median is the best choice. Although the mode provides the same value as the median in this case, it would generally be biased when the intensity distribution was multimodal.

In estimating the true signal value, it is necessary to reduce the effect of nonspecific fluorescence, such as the autofluorescence of the glass slides. For most analysis calculations, the background intensity should be subtracted from the signal intensity before any ratio calculations are performed. The method for determining the background intensity can vary, depending on the quality of the arrays and the spacing between individual spots. The same measurements discussed earlier, such as mean, median, mode, and total, can be used to compute the background.

Further, one can also compute the standard deviation of the background intensities that can be used to determine the reliability of the measurement. If the standard deviation is high, the background is nonuniform and chances are that part of the signal is accounted for as background. If the spot spacing is too small, it may be advisable to compute a measurement value based on the grouping of several, or even all spots. The noise in the background region will ultimately determine how well one can resolve whether the signal is significantly above background. The noise is estimated by computing the standard deviation of the pixels in the background region. A common method for establishing signal threshold is to add one or two times the standard deviation to the background value. A spot with a measurement larger than this value is likely to be a true signal.

### Importance of Quality Measurements

An important step in processing microarray images is to assess the reliability of the data obtained and to report the problems in the images that may be arising from the array fabrication process and experiments. These tasks may be performed by a human operator or by image-processing algorithms. The importance of these tasks needs to be emphasized. Without assessing the reliability of the data, the conclusions drawn from analyzing such data may be misleading. Very often such errors can lead to following a false hypothesis or missing important findings.

The reliability of the data is affected by multiple factors, ranging from problems in array fabrication to problems in image processing. In high-throughput gene expression analysis systems, the reliability assessment needs to be done by a software system. Figure 3.7 shows an example of how quality measurements can be used to improve the reliability of the data. The data were obtained from an image file processed by a fully automatic image-analysis system. The coefficient of variation (CV) (standard deviation/mean) was 27%. Using spot size as the quality measurement, we discarded about 25% of the spots that were excessively large or small. The coefficient of variation was reduced to 18.5%, suggesting an improvement of the reliability of the data after weeding out low-quality spots.

### Operational Modes and Their Effect on Data Reliability

An aspect common to all array processing techniques is the extent of reliability, repeatability, and variance in measurements. So far,

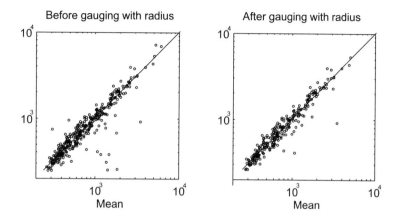

**Figure 3.7** The reliability improvement following quality control. The figures are scatter plots of the mean values obtained from duplicated spots. The axes are the mean pixel intensity values. The left figure consists of data from all the spots in the image. The right figure plots 75% of the spots in the left figure. The 25% discarded spots have excessively large or small radii. The coefficient of variance is 27% for the left figure and 18.6% for the right, a reduction of 30%.

it has been very difficult to validate the different processing algorithms because of the large amounts of data needed to ensure sufficient statistical analysis of the measurements reported. As with sequencing, the best comparisons and measures of reliability can only be made when large datasets containing significant repetitions and overlapping data are freely available.

We performed a series of dilution studies in which the same clone was repeated on a single $10 \times 15$ array. The Cy3-dUTP was incorporated into 35-mer oligonucleotides. A sample image from the study is shown in figure 3.8. The array was scanned sequentially six times using the same scan settings. Photobleaching was estimated as 0.6% per scan. The expression strength was measured using the processing techniques discussed in the earlier sections.

The images were processed using five different techniques, each of which is:

- *Fully automatic.* Spot finding was performed automatically simply by providing the array configuration and the expected size of

**Figure 3.8** A sample from the dilution series study.

the spots. The spots were automatically adjusted both for size and location. The combined segmentation technique was used and the difference between the signal and background means was used to compute the expression strength.

- *Semiautomatic with trimmed measurements.* Spot finding was performed by manually specifying the spot locations and finally updating the position based on local neighborhoods. The method of trimmed measurements was used to segment the signal and background pixels.
- *Semiautomatic with Mann–Whitney test.* This was the same as above, except the Mann–Whitney test was used to segment the signal and background pixels.
- *Manual.* The spots were placed manually and the segmentation was based on the signal inside the circle and the background outside, but was bounded by another circle of a fixed diameter.

The processing was performed on all the images and was repeated ten times to check the introduction of variability due to user bias. To compare the measurements obtained, each of the datasets was first normalized across the repeated spots. Each image

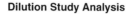

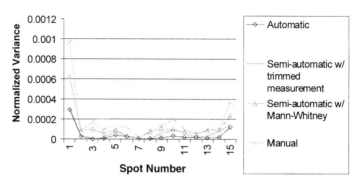

**Figure 3.9** Variance estimated between different processing techniques based on a series of Cy3-dUTP dilution studies.

had 15 dilutions where each spot was repeated 10 times. By normalizing and factoring the photobleaching, we were able to eliminate the variability caused by spotting and uneven distribution of the mRNA. Next, the resulting measurements were normalized across the repeated processing measurements so that the expression strength had a mean of 0 and a standard deviation of 1. Now, by examining the variation within the normalized data, we could assess the reliability of the measured values based on the different processing techniques.

Figure 3.9 shows a plot of the spots' normalized expression strengths against the variance that was due to different processing techniques. As shown, the lowest variance is seen in fully automated processing followed by semiautomatic with trimmed measurements, semiautomatic with the Mann–Whitney test, and finally the manual mode. It is clear that the automated mode is much more flexible because it is able to account for variability in the data more efficiently by quantifying the correct signal, background, and contaminated pixels.

Also noticeable is the significant increase in variance while processing in a nonautomated mode as the expression strength increases. This observation suggests that the automatic removal of contaminated pixels and the combined spatial and intensity estimation of signal and background pixels results in improved differencing between the signal and background measurements. It is fairly evident that automated processing with statistical measurement and quality assessment may be optimal for reliable high-throughput microarray analysis.

## Data Analysis and Visualization Techniques

The image-processing and analysis step produces a large number of quantified gene expression values. The data typically represent thousands or tens of thousands of gene expression levels across multiple experiments. To make sense of this much information, use of various visualization and statistical analysis techniques is unavoidable. One of the typical microarray data analysis goals is to find statistically significant up- or downregulated genes—in other words, outliers or "interestingly" behaving genes in the data (Heyer et al., 1999). Another possible goal would be to find functional groupings of genes by discovering similarities or dissimilarities among gene expression profiles, or predicting the biochemical and physiological pathways of previously uncharacterized genes (Hilsenbeck et al., 1999). In the following sections, we discuss visualization approaches and algorithms implementing various multivariate techniques that could help realize the above-mentioned goals and could help solve the needs of the microarray research community.

### Scatter Plot

Probably the simplest analysis tool for visualization of microarray data is the scatter plot. In a scatter plot, each point represents the expression value of a gene in two experiments—one assigned to the x-axis and the other to the y-axis, as shown in figure 3.10. In

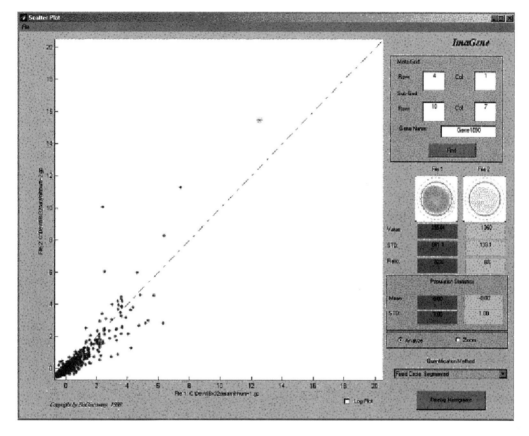

**Figure 3.10**  Scatter plot of two experiments. Every point in the plot represents a single gene. The position of the point on the graph shows the expression value of the gene in the two experiments shown on the axes.

such a plot, genes with equal expression values in both experiments would line up on the identity line (diagonal). Genes that are differentially expressed will be plotted away from the diagonal. The further away a gene is plotted from the identity line, the larger is the difference between its expression in one experiment and another. The absolute strength of the expression levels can be readily visualized in this plot since the higher expression values are plotted farther away from the origin.

## Principal Component Analysis

It is easy to see how the scatter plot is an ideal tool for comparing the expression profile of genes in two experiments. Three experiments could be plotted and compared in a three-dimensional scatter plot. Three-dimensional plots can be rendered and manipulated on a computer screen. However, when more than three experiments are to be analyzed and compared, the simple scatter plot cannot be used. In the case of twenty experiments, for example, we cannot draw a twenty-dimensional plot. Fortunately, there are mathematical techniques available for reducing dimensionality, such as principal component analysis (PCA) (Duda and Hart, 1973; Johnson and Wichern, 1998; Raychaudhuri et al., 2000), in which high-dimensional space can be projected down to two or three dimensions. The goal of all dimensionality reduction methods is to perform this operation while preserving most or all the variances of the original data set. In other words, if two points are relatively "close" to one another in the high-dimensional space, they will be relatively close in the lower dimensional space as well. In general, it is not possible to maintain this relationship perfectly. Imagine that a three-dimensional spherical orange peel is made flat on the two-dimentional surface of a table. Most of the points lying on the surface of the orange peel keep their relationship to their neighbors. However, to flatten it, we must tear the orange peel in several places, thus breaking the neighboring relationship between some points on the peel.

PCA is a method that attempts to preserve the neighboring relationships as much as possible. Figure 3.11 is a three-dimensional plot of 600 genes in 21 experiments, indicating the position of all 600 genes with respect to the first three principal components. Each principal component is made up of a linear combination (summation) of all the 600 genes, each weighted by a different value.

This multivariate technique is frequently used to provide a compact representation of large amounts of data by finding the axes (principal components) on which the data vary the most. In prin-

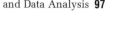

**Figure 3.11** Principal component analysis on 600 genes across 21 experiments. Gene scores are plotted on the first three principal components.

cipal component analysis, the coefficients for the variables are chosen so that the first component explains the maximum amount of variance in the data. The second principal component is perpendicular to the first one and explains the maximum of the residual variance. The third component is perpendicular to the first two and explains the maximum residual variance. This process is continued until all the variance in the data is explained.

The linear combination of gene expression levels on the first three principal components could easily be visualized in a 3D plot (figure 3.11). This method, like the scatter plot, provides an easy way of finding outliers in the data (genes that behave differently than most of the genes across a set of experiments). It can also reveal clusters of genes that behave similarly across different experiments.

Principal component analysis can also be performed on the experiments to find out possible groupings and/or outliers of experiments. In this case, every point plotted in the 3D graph would represent a unique microarray experiment. Points that are placed close to one another represent experiments that have similar expression patterns. Recent findings show that this method should be able to even detect moderate-sized alterations in gene expression (Hilsenbeck et al., 1999). In general, principal component analysis provides a rather practical approach to data reduction, visualization, and identification of unusually behaving, outlier genes and/or experiments.

### Parallel Coordinate Planes

Two and three-dimensional scatter plots and principal component analysis plots are ideal for detecting significantly up- or down-regulated genes across a set of experiments. These methods, however, do not provide an easy way of visualizing progression of gene expression over several experiments. These types of questions usually come up in time series experiments where, for instance, gene expression is measured at 2-hour intervals. The important question in this case is how gene expression values vary over the duration of the entire experiment.

The parallel coordinate planes plotting technique is an ideal visualization tool to answer these types of questions. With this method, experiments are ordered on the x-axis and expression values are plotted on the y-axis. All genes in a given experiment are plotted at the same location on the x-axis, while their y locations are varied. Another experiment is plotted at another x location in the plane. Typically, the progression of time would be mapped into the x-axis by having higher x values for experiments done at a later time. By connecting the expression values for the same genes in the different experiments, one can obtain a very intuitive way of depicting the progression of gene expression.

### Cluster Analysis

Another frequently asked question related to microarrays is that of finding groups of genes with similar expression profiles across a number of experiments. The most commonly used multivariate technique to find such groups is cluster analysis. Essentially, these techniques arrive at an ordering of the data, which groups (clusters) genes with similar expression patterns closer to each other. These techniques can help establish functional groupings of genes or predict the biochemical and physiological pathways of previously uncharacterized genes.

The clustering method that is most frequently used in the literature for finding groups in microarray data is hierarchical clustering (Duda and Hart, 1973; Eisen et al., 1998). This method attempts to group genes and/or experiments in small clusters and then group these clusters into higher-level clusters and so on. As a result of this clustering or grouping process, a tree of connectivity of observations emerges that can easily be visualized as dendrograms. For gene expression data, not only the grouping of genes, but also the grouping of experiments might also be important. When both are considered, it becomes easy to simultaneously search for patterns in gene expression profiles and across many different experimental conditions, as shown in figure 3.12. For example, a group of genes behaving similarly (e.g., all upregulated) can be seen in a particular group of experiments.

Every colored block in the middle panel of figure 3.12 represents the expression value of a gene in an experiment. The 600 genes are plotted horizontally and the 6 experiments are plotted vertically. The color code for gene expression is located in the lower-right corner. The dendrogram for genes is located just above the color-coded expression values, with one arm connected to every gene in the study. The dendrogram for experiments is on the left, showing the grouping of the 21 experiments in the study.

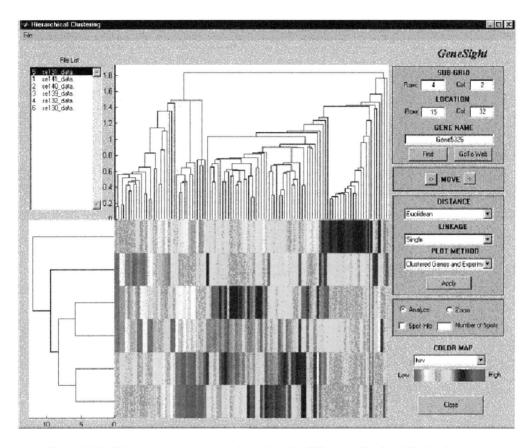

**Figure 3.12** Color-coded gene expression values for 600 genes (horizontally) in six experiments (vertically). Simultaneous clustering of genes and experiments is shown by the top and left side dendrograms, respectively.

Although hierarchical clustering is currently a commonly employed way of finding groupings in the data, other, nonhierarchical (k-means) methods are likely to gain more popularity in the future. This is largely due to the rapidly growing amounts of data and the ever-increasing average experiment size. A common characteristic of nonhierarchical approaches is to provide sufficient clustering without having to create the full distance or similarity matrix, while minimizing the number of scans of the whole data set.

**APPLIED BIOSYSTEMS**

### Data Normalization and Transformation

It is important to realize that even with the most powerful statistical methods, the success of an analysis is crucially dependent on the "cleanness" and statistical properties of the data. Essentially, the two questions to ask before even starting any analysis are:

1. Does the variation in the data represent true variation in expression values, or is it contaminated by differences in expression caused by experimental variability?
2. Are the data "well behaving" in terms of meeting the underlying assumptions of the statistical analysis techniques that are applied to it?

It is easy to appreciate the importance of the first point. The significance of the second one comes from the fact that most multivariate analysis techniques are based on underlying assumptions such as normality and homoscedasticity. If these assumptions are not met, at least approximately, then the whole statistical analysis could be distorted, and statistical tests might be invalid. Fortunately, there are a variety of statistical techniques available to help us answer "yes" to the above questions. These are normalization (standardization) and transformations.

Normalization can help us separate true variation in expression values from differences that are due to experimental variability. This step is necessary since it is quite possible that because of the complexity of creating, hybridizing, scanning, and quantifying microarrays, variation originating from the experimental process may contaminate the data. During a typical microarray experiment, many different variables and parameters can possibly change, differentially affecting the measured expression levels. Among these are slide quality, pin quality, amount of DNA spotted, accuracy of arraying device, dye characteristics, scanner quality, and quantification software characteristics, just to name a few. The various methods of normalization aim at removing or at least minimizing expression differences that are due to variability in any of these types of conditions.

As discussed here, the various transformation methods all aim at changing the variance and distribution properties of the data in such a way that it would be closer in meeting the underlying assumptions of the statistical techniques applied to it in the analysis phase. The most common requirements of statistical techniques are for the data to have homologous variance (homoscedasticity) and normal distribution (normality). In the following section, several popular ways of normalizing and transforming microarray data are discussed.

NORMALIZATION OF THE DATA

One of the most popular ways to control for spotted DNA quantity and other slide characteristics is to do a type of local normalization by using two channels (e.g., red and green) in the experiment. For example, a Cy5 (red)-labeled probe could be used as a control prepared from a mixture of cDNA samples or from normal cDNA. Then a Cy3 (green)-labeled experimental probe could be prepared from cDNA extracted from a tumor tissue. The normalized expression values for every gene would then be calculated as the ratio of experimental and control expression.

This method can obviously eliminate a great portion of experimental variation by providing every spot (gene) in the experiment with its own control. Developing on these ideas, three-channel experiments are under way in which one channel serves as control for the other two. In this case, the expression values of both experimental channels would be divided by the same control value.

In addition to the local normalization method described above, global methods are also available in the form of "control" spots on the slide. Based on a set of these control spots, it is possible to control for global variation in overall slide quality or scanning differences.

The above procedures describe some physical measures in terms of spotting characteristics that one can take to normalize the microarray data. However, even after the most careful two- or more channel spotting with the use of control spots, it is still possible

A                                          B

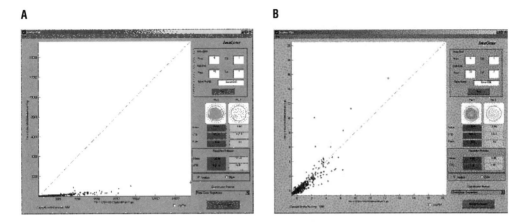

**Figure 3.13** (*A*) Scatter plot of two experiments in which the signal values are significantly stronger in one file than in the other. (*B*) The same data as in (*A*) after normalization.

that undesired experimental variation will contaminate the expression data. On the other hand, it is also possible that all or some of the physical normalization techniques are missing from the experiment, in which case it is even more important to find other ways of normalization.

Fortunately for both of these scenarios, additional statistics-based normalization methods are available to further clean up the data. As an example, the situation can occur where, for the same set of genes, expression values in one experiment are consistently and significantly different from those in another experiment—perhaps owing to quality differences between the slides, or the printing or scanning process, or possibly some other factor. This is evident from the scatter plot seen in figure 3.13.

It might be very misleading to compare the expression values of the two files plotted in figure 3.13A without any normalization. In figure 3.13B, the same data are plotted after normalization. Notice that most of the gene expressions now lie on the identity line, as would be expected for two experiments on the same set of genes.

TRANSFORMATION OF THE DATA

Although there are many different data transforms available, the most frequently used procedure in the microarray literature is to take the logarithm of the quantified expression values (Hilsenbeck et al., 1999; Eisen et al., 1998). An often-cited reason for applying such a transform is to equalize variability in the typically wildly varying raw expression scores. If the expression value was calculated as a ratio of experimental over control conditions, then an additional effect of the log transform will be to equate up- and downregulation by the same amount in absolute value scores ($\log_{10} 2 = 0.3$ and $\log_{10} 0.5 = -0.3$). Another important side effect of the log transform is to bring the distribution of the data closer to normal. Having reasonable grounds of meeting the normality and homoscedasticity assumptions after the log transform, the use of a variety of parametric statistical analysis methods is also much more justifiable (Johnson and Wichern, 1998).

As shown in the left panel of figure 3.14, without the log transform we get a very peaked distribution of the data, with a very long tail. This distribution is very far from normal, which violates the

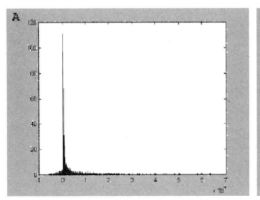 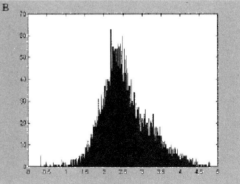

**Figure 3.14** Histograms of the previously cited gene expression data (600 genes × 21 experiments). The x-axis indicates the expression values and the y-axis shows the number of genes with a particular gene expression level. The left and right panels show the data before and after the log transform, respectively.

assumptions made by many standard parametric statistical analysis methods. The distribution of the log-transformed data in the right panel is visibly much closer to that of the normal distribution, which could also be verified by a simple normality test. Certainly other types of transforms could also be investigated. In fact, the choice of transformation should be dependent on the one that brings the data closest to the requirements of homogeneity of variance and normal distribution (Johnson and Wichern, 1998). It turns out that for most microarray expression data, the log transform provides the best solution.

## Summary

Although microarray-based analysis and exploration faces technical hurdles, there is room for optimism. There is a potential for unprecedented throughput with a high degree of accuracy. Microarray technology is in its infancy, and further improvements will ensure that it matures into an even more powerful analytical tool for accurate and high-throughput genomic analysis. Common standards will be required before investigators can meaningfully extract and combine data, which will have to be stored in databases that can be effectively mined. Despite the early stage of development of large-scale gene expression monitoring systems and methods, this new technology has already proven exceptionally useful in expanding our knowledge of even well-understood aspects of cellular biology.

From an information-processing perspective, microarray technology aids the researcher in transforming and supplementing available genetic and cellular data to obtain useful information about gene expression and ultimately cellular biology. In this chapter we have described the various issues that are involved in this process, starting from the data management and tracking involved in production of the arrays, to the analysis of high-density array images, and finally to the analysis of the massive amount of data generated by microarray experiments. However, we must also realize that there remain many challenges in addressing the software needs of the microarray technology. High-quality data and the accuracy of data extracted from microarray images form the basis of a well-designed software system.

## Acknowledgments

The authors would like to thank Dr. Bruce Hoff, Mr. James Park, and Mr. Jing-Ying Chen for their creative ideas and help during the development of the algorithms used in the writing of this chapter. We would also like to thank Dr. Jeff Gregg at the University of California, Davis School of Medicine, for his input on the genomic experimentation techniques and providing us with the dilution study series. Finally, we would also like to thank Mr. Jeff Smith for his help with analysis of the experiments discussed.

## References

Beulieu JM and Goldberg M (1989). Hierarchy in picture segmentation: A stepwise optimization approach. *IEEE Trans PAMI* 11(2): 150–63.

Chen Y, Dougherty ER, and Bittner ML (1997). Ratio-based decisions and the quantitative analysis of cDNA microarray images. *J Biomedical Optics* 2(4): 364–74.

Duda RO and Hart PE (1973). *Pattern Classification and Scene Analysis*. J. Wiley, New York.

Eisen MB, Spellman PT, Brown PO, and Botstein D (1998). Cluster analysis and display of genome-wide expression patterns. *Proc Natl Acad Sci USA* 95: 14863–8.

Haralick RM (1979). Statistical and structural approaches to texture. *Proc IEEE* 67: 786–804.

Heyer LJ, Kruglyak S, and Yooseph S (1999). Exploring expression data: Identification and analysis of coexpressed genes. *Genome Res* 9: 1106–15.

Hilsenbeck SG, Friedrichs WE, Schiff R, O'Connell P, Hansen RK, Osborne CK, and Fuqua SAW (1999). Statistical analysis of array expression data as applied to the problem of tamoxifen resistance. *J Natl Cancer Inst* 91(5): 453–9.

Johnson RA and Wichern DA (1998). *Applied Multivariate Statistical Analysis*. Prentice Hall, Upper Saddle River, NJ.

Pal NR and Pal SK (1993). A review on image segmentation techniques. *Pattern Recognition* 26(9): 1277–94.

Price K (1984). Image segmentation: A comment on studies in global and local histogram-guided relaxation algorithms. *IEEE Trans PAMI* 6(2): 247–9.

Raychaudhuri S, Stuart JM, and Altman RB (2000). Principal components analysis to summarize microarray experiments: application to sporulation time series. Presented at Pacific Symposium on Biocomputing, Oahu, Hawaii. *Proceedings of Pacific Symposium on Biocomputing*, vol. 5, pp. 452–63.

Shah S and Aggarwal JK (1998). Multiple feature integration for robust object localization. Presented at the Computer Society Conference on Computer Vision and Pattern Recognition, Santa Barbara, CA, June 1988. *Proceedings of Computer Society Conference on Computer Vision and Pattern Recognition*, pp. 765–71.

Shah S and Aggarwal JK (1997a). A Bayesian segmentation framework for textured visual images. Presented at the Computer Society Conference on Computer Vision and Pattern Recognition, San Juan, Puerto Rico, June 1997. *Proceedings of Computer Society Conference on Computer Vision and Pattern Recognition*, pp. 1014–20.

Shah S and Aggarwal JK (1997b). Object recognition and performance bounds. *Lecture Notes in Computer Science: Image Analysis and Processing*. Del Bimbo A, ed. Springer-Verlag, New York, pp. 343–60.

Spann M and Nieminen A (1988). Adaptive Gaussian weighted filtering for image segmentation. *Pattern Recognition Lett* 8: 251–5.

# 4 Statistical Inference in Array Genomics

Robert Nadon, Erik Woody, Peide Shi, Nezar Rghei, Hermann Hubschle, Edward Susko, and Peter Ramm

The most dedicated users of array technology have been industrial drug discovery programs seeking tractable drug targets among disease-linked proteins. Typically the hypotheses are of the kind: "Expression in genes A and B is elevated under disease entity X," and "Disease-related genes A and B exhibit normal levels of expression following administration of compound Y." While the technologies for conducting experiments relevant to such hypotheses are readily available, the analytical methods used in hypothesis testing lag behind the paradigms for array creation, processing, and detection. That is, technologies for running array studies are more sophisticated than the methods for making sense of them. Analytical methods are therefore under intense investigation.

The need for rigorous analytical methods may be particularly pressing in neuroscience applications, which have already produced massive amounts of data. Neuroscience hypotheses might be summarized as: "A particular expression pattern is linked to neural state X." For X, we could substitute anything from receptor kinetics to process elaboration to bipolar depression. These phenomena are less well defined than the protein pathways that are usually linked to expression values. Moreover, next-stage experiments are complex and likely to involve living tissues or organisms. For these reasons, poorly qualified expression findings can be particularly costly. In this chapter we discuss some of the general issues affecting array analysis and describe a new, sensitive method for applying inferential statistics to expression arrays.

## General Analytical Issues

### Nonstatistical Approaches

Early approaches to array analysis used arbitrary thresholds to discriminate between meaningful and nonmeaningful expression differences. Very small fold-changes in expression (e.g., 1.2 : 1) would be considered to be chance observations. By contrast, fold-changes greater than some specified amount (e.g., two- or threefold) would be judged to reflect "true" differences (see, e.g., Bassett et al., 1999).

Threshold methods attempted to incorporate corrections for systematic error (see later discussion) by referencing each spot value to some internal reference or set of references. For example, relative to a reference gene, a spot may show a 2:1 ratio when measured at time 1, a 2.8:1 ratio when measured at time 2, and so on (Ermolaeva et al., 1998; Schena et al., 1996). Threshold approaches, however, have deficiencies.

Threshold values and assessments of confidence in those values (e.g., why threefold is acceptable and twofold is not) are established according to the beliefs of the individual researcher, and cannot be validated in formal ways. Moreover, there is no single threshold value that is sensitive across the entire range of expression values. Rather, the optimal threshold varies with the random error present in the data. Random error, in turn, varies with the intensity of the signals making up the ratio. That is, a threefold change based on high signal levels will have a different confidence interval than another threefold change based on signal levels near background. A fixed threshold can tend to detract from experimental sensitivity with high confidence data points, while it generates too many false positives with low confidence data points.

In addition, many of the early informal rules for analyzing array data were developed using raw scale measurements. A consensus has emerged that the appropriate metric for array data is a log scale (any base). Log-transformed array data tend to be normally distributed, and this property makes the data appropriate for parametric statistical testing (e.g., *t*-tests, analyses of variance). A log transformation also makes the random error component less dependent on signal intensity. One desirable consequence of this is a concomitant reduction in the number of extreme (and spurious) ratio values because the influence of incorporating a small expression value in the numerator or denominator of a ratio is reduced.

## Use of Hypothesis Testing Methods

Array users have debated whether a hypothesis-driven approach is too limiting in the face of the vast numbers of data points arising from array studies. Some favor an approach to data analysis (and to publishing) that is as free from a priori constraints as possible (Brown and Botstein, 1999; Goodman, 1999). Others suggest that in silico and in vitro methodologies have become efficient enough to allow parallel experimental validation of expression "hits." It is more common, however, for array researchers to advocate the classical approach of conducting initial exploratory work that is followed by hypothesis-driven cross-validation studies (Lander, 1999; Staudt, 2000).

Hypothesis-testing approaches have at least two advantages. They provide (1) a self-correcting mechanism for false positive errors generated by unconstrained exploratory data analytical methods and (2) procedures that are readily standardized across laboratories and array paradigms.

## Replicates

The earliest array studies did not use replicates, prompting the development of singleton methods to determine random measurement error (Chen et al., 1997). Practical arguments favoring the use of singleton measurements usually relate to conservation of costly and/or rare resources. It has also been argued that when array data are checked using low-throughput methods (Cole et al., 1999), external validity is established with reference to biology rather than inherent properties of the array. There are many more data points originating from arrays, however, than can be checked efficiently. Moreover, even the most careful post hoc validation of positive observations will fail to control false negative errors.

The view that replicates are required is becoming widespread (Lee et al., 2000) and most array users recognize the advantages of replicates. Averages of expression values can be obtained, thereby improving measurement reliability. The random error associated with single measurements is larger than that associated with measurements averaged across replicates. As a consequence, single measurements have wider confidence intervals and are less sensitive to differences in expression.

Replicates can also improve data quality through outlier detection procedures. Such procedures are essential to the current state of the array art because few arrays are extremely clean. Replicates allow us to specify whether unusual observations are due to errors of some sort (e.g., dust artifact) or reflect true differences in expression. The issue of outlier rejection is most pressing in high-throughput applications, when there is no possibility of visually scanning all the data to perform subjective artifact removal. In addition, in a new and rapidly changing field, there is something to be said for using methods that follow standard scientific practice. We believe that the publication standards of most journals will soon require replicates.

**Clipping and Saturation Effects**

Scanners are often set so that there are clipped measurements at the low end of the detector dynamic range (floor effect) and saturated measurements at the high end of the range (ceiling effect). In most cases, this is an elementary source of error that can be easily corrected at the data acquisition stage.

### Data Mining and Inferential Analyses

Data mining and statistical inference methods provide different but complementary information. Data mining methods separate large data sets into more manageable groupings (clusters) and thereby help to visualize complex relationships in an exploratory fashion. By contrast, statistical inference techniques provide confirmatory tests of specific hypotheses and their associated probability values. A schematic view of how the two methods complement each other is shown in figure 4.1.

The exploratory nature of data mining makes it difficult to establish which mining results reflect "true" relationships and which reflect "chance." It is a common observation that different mining methods lead to different results with the same data, illustrating the difficulty in justifying the use of a particular mining technique. The field is complex; there are no well-established standards; and there is the possibility that selection of a mining method can be affected by the expectations of the researcher. For these reasons, experimental methodologists favor validating data-mining results with inferential methods before making more definitive conclusions.

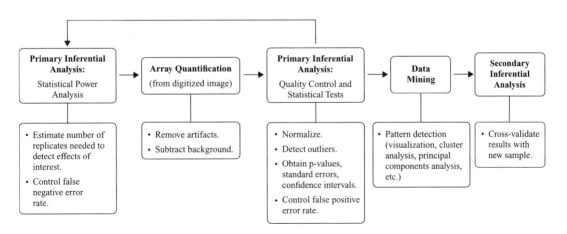

**Figure 4.1** Schematic view of array data analysis.

One way to do this is to study known pathways or interactions. The results of various mining techniques can then be compared to determine which method provides the best "prediction" of the known results. The best technique in one data analysis context, however, may not be the best when applied in another, less well-understood context. Along these lines, existing data-mining algorithms have not always been satisfactory when applied to array genomics questions, prompting the recent focus on adapting standard methods and developing new ones for application to array data (Bassett et al., 1999; Brown and Botstein, 1999; Claverie, 1999; Sherlock, 2000). In the final analysis, inferential cross-validation of data-mining output to a new sample (secondary inferential analysis) provides the best assurance that initial data-mining results reflect meaningful effects.

Statistical inference procedures can also be beneficial before mining analyses (primary inferential analysis). They can be used when there are a priori experimental hypotheses (e.g., "cell line A expresses gene X at a level different from cell line B") and can also be used to perform "shotgun" testing. ("Which probes hybridize differently to lines A and B?") The result of an inferential analysis is a list of all the genes, with attribution of statistical significance to just a few. Contrary to data mining, inferential techniques can control false positive error rates, estimate the probability of false negative errors, and assign probability values, confidence intervals, standard errors, and so forth to expression comparisons.

Primary inferential analyses provide objective information about differential expression at the level of individual genes and, as such, can stand alone. They can also be used to improve data quality for subsequent data-mining analyses. Relative to prevalent standards, the quality of information derived from expression arrays can be improved in at least four ways by using primary statistical inference methods:

1. Power analysis can be used to estimate the number of replicates needed to achieve a desired level of sensitivity for detecting a specified effect size, thereby minimizing false negative errors.

2. Outlier detection can eliminate poorly reproduced expression values that bias the measurement of both expression intensities and random error estimates.

3. Standard statistical indices ($p$-values, standard errors, confidence intervals) provide formal objective rules for making judgments about differential expression.

4. False positive errors can be minimized with various multiple test correction procedures (e.g., Bonferroni method).

## The Nature of Error

As with other scientific data, array data should be reproducible from specimen to specimen, study to study, and lab to lab. Reproducibility is a necessary (but not sufficient) condition for biological validity. The types of errors that adversely affect reproducibility can be categorized as errors of measurement and errors of inference.

### Errors of Measurement

We obtain an understanding of reproducibility by estimating the error in a measurement. There are two classes of measurement error that affect array data: systematic error and random error. Systematic error refers to differences in background, labeling intensity, and other factors that cause overall differences among arrays. We try to correct systematic error by removing it. Random error reflects noise that obscures the precision of our measurement. Noise can be reduced by various image-processing and numerical procedures, but it cannot be removed entirely. Rather, we use the magnitude of random error as a key criterion against which each observation of expression is compared.

### Systematic Error

A measured value is unbiased (has no systematic error) if it does not over- or underestimate the "true" population value. Typical sources of experimental bias lie within array processing and within the detection paradigm. These errors are corrected by procedures called "background subtraction" and "normalization." Both forms of correction are used in almost every array study.

BACKGROUND SUBTRACTION

Within arrays, background contributes to measured signal values in what is assumed to be a linear additive fashion. Therefore, the biasing effect of background is corrected by subtraction. Background varies from point to point across an array, and estimates are typically obtained from areas adjacent to spots (e.g., circular regions surrounding each spot), from negative control spots, from a mean of all nonspot areas, and so on. In general, a successful background correction is one that does not result in the loss of low-intensity spot values (by subtracting too large a background estimate), but which removes almost all of the nonsignal component. It is critical that background be removed prior to any subsequent analysis. Fortunately, many array quantification software packages now include effective corrections for background so that background bias is not a major factor in data analysis.

NORMALIZATION

Other sources of systematic error arise within the signal itself and can be more difficult to correct. Concentration errors are those which arise when label intensity is not linearly related to hybridization. For example, various chemical and physical processes become self-limiting at high concentrations (e.g., self-quenching), and this can compress the upper range of response in a hybridization measurement system. Ideally, we would like to calibrate our arrays so that such errors are accounted for.

Methods used to calibrate hybridization to label concentrations include exposing spiked standards with each array and then fitting a curve to the standards. This is normal practice in many types of quantitative imaging (e.g., quantitative autoradiography), where precisely calibrated standards are readily available.

The creation of representative standards for hybridization studies, however, is particularly complex. The difficulty lies in knowing the extent to which label intensity reflects absolute message levels (Duggan et al., 1999). As a result, even calibrated expression arrays provide only relative measurements (one spot is specified as 50% brighter than another one, instead of specifying 150 labeled molecules vs. 100). While standards can help to reduce severe nonlinearities, hybridization measurements can retain a biasing component after calibration. This problem is most marked when two fluors (one used as an internal control) are used to construct ratios. The magnitude of the ratio will be biased by what is usually a fluor-specific relation between intensity and hybridization (Bartosiewicz et al., 2000). Compounding the difficulties in multicolor arrays, fluorescent dyes are different in mean brightness, and exhibit a differing background offset (Geiss et al., 2000).

In addition, there are many other biasing factors that affect array measurements. Target accessibility is affected by variations in the absorbency of discrete nylon membranes of the same make (Perret et al., 1998). Even the time of day that arrays are processed (Lander, 1999) and variations in washing procedures (Shalon et al., 1996) have been cited as systematic error factors.

These various systematic errors are proportional to signal intensity and are corrected by normalization. Normalization procedures typically divide signal intensities by a reference value, derived in various alternative ways:

1. *Mean of all spots on the array.* This brings the average intensity of the normalized spots to a value of 1. This procedure assumes that most genes are not differentially expressed across conditions.
2. *Subset of spots.* A subset of probes is laid down (e.g., housekeeping genes) whose expression levels are assumed to be unrelated to the independent variable (across conditions). Early enthusiasm for housekeeping genes has waned, and the search for appropriate normalization references is continuing (Eickhoff et al., 1999; Ermolaeva et al., 1998).

3. *Spiked spots.* Spots containing known concentrations of a heterologous probe are used as a reference.

It should be remembered that normalization addresses only the relative accuracy of observations. Remaining extraneous factors (such as the concentration error described earlier) can continue to detract from the linearity of measurements. Measurement non-linearity makes comparisons across experiments or laboratories much more difficult than they should be, and the development of optimal calibration standards remains a high priority.

Until the field settles on standard methods for correcting systematic error, informal procedures will make implicit (and potentially incorrect) assumptions about the structure of the data. In doing so, they are subject to measurement bias. For example, normalizing each spot value to the mean of a reference set yields error properties (see the next section for why error properties are important) that are different from those of a procedure that normalizes by first taking a log of each value and then subtracting the mean of the reference set. Similarly, using housekeeping genes that respond to the independent variable or failing to remove outliers within the reference set before normalization biases error correction.

Finally, the usual practice treats the normalization reference value as a constant, failing to take into account the random error associated with the reference. The confidence bounds around a reference value based on a small number of replicates in particular will tend to be large, diminishing its value as a reference. (Assuming 10–15% variation, 5–10 reference replicates should provide sufficient measurement precision for most applications.) A formal statistical model, applied in standard ways, is needed to allow optimal and verifiable correction of systematic error. We discuss such a model in later sections.

## Random Error

Once systematic error has been removed, any remaining measurement error is, in theory, random. Random error reflects the expected statistical variation in a measured value. Low random error corresponds to high precision (an ability to detect small differences) and is indexed by highly reproducible measurements. Ideally, random error should be estimated from the variation displayed by replicate values.

That successful use of standard statistical tests is highly dependent upon good estimates of random error is recognized in the genomics community (Bassett et al., 1999). A particular problem in array studies, however, is that the sample sizes are small. Few array users have more than four replicates, and many have only two. Unfortunately, estimates of random error based on small samples are themselves very variable, making standard statistical tests imprecise and impractical. It is not surprising, therefore, that early approaches to analysis of array data were either explicitly nonstatistical or circumvented usual statistical practice.

It has been suggested that the most challenging aspects of presenting expression data involve the quantification and qualification of expression values using standard statistical significance tests and confidence intervals (Bassett et al., 1999). The problem, of course, is that any transcript must be present in sufficient replicates to be suited to standard statistical tests. Without this, standard statistical indices (e.g., confidence intervals, outlier delineation) and parametric statistical tests are both insensitive and suspect.

To illustrate the problem, consider a population of repeated measurements of a specific gene. The central limit theorem informs us that the sampling distribution of means obtained from this population approaches normality as the sample size increases, whatever the shape of the population distribution. This is an important consideration for the usual parametric statistical tests, which assume normality of the sampling distribution. With relatively large sample sizes ($> 10$, for example), we can be reasonably assured that the sampling distribution is approximately normal, even if the parent population is not. This assurance diminishes, however, when sample sizes are very small and/or when the parent distribution is highly skewed.

Violation of the normality assumption with small samples sizes makes parametric tests inappropriate for making inferences about differential expression. Moreover, in usual circumstances, there is simply no way of knowing whether the normality assumption has been met. Nonparametric alternatives (e.g., Mann–Whitney U test, Wilcoxon's Matched-Pairs Signed-Ranks Test) are available, but are too insensitive to detect any but the largest changes when sample sizes are very small.

OUTLIERS
Outliers are unusually small or large values that differ from other replicates obtained under the same conditions. Because the conditions are the same, outliers commonly reflect an artifact of some kind (dust, bits of probe sprayed about) rather than biology, and are deleted from the analysis.

Outliers can be detected during both quantification of the array images and subsequent statistical analysis of the array data. The methods used at these two stages are quite different. During image analysis, pixel-based tests are used to search out deviant areas of the image (artifacts). Examples of pixel-based outlier identification would include spots containing bright bits with dustlike features, spots with large pixel-to-pixel variability, or spots that exhibit poor signal-to-noise characteristics in comparison with local background.

During statistical analysis, outliers are detected on the basis of their deviation from other replicates. Again, we have two issues arising from the small sample numbers: (1) A single outlier can seriously skew data interpretation of a small sample and (2) estimates of random error are insensitive, so detection of deviant variation is also insensitive.

Without an accurate random error estimate, outlier detection is based on arbitrary rules. A typical case (Perret et al., 1998) compared sets of two replicates after normalization. Any replicate set that showed a greater than twofold difference between its members was regarded as an outlier. Although this type of approach is preferable to no outlier detection at all, there is no way of optimizing outlier rejection according to the actual properties of the array without a probability-based statistical model. Informal methods will also tend to vary in effectiveness because random error varies among arrays while the informal method does not (or varies arbitrarily). For example, a twofold difference between replicates may be large or small, depending upon the amount of random error.

These types of measurement error and quality control problems compound the difficulties of making inferences about differential expression outside of a formal statistical model. This in turn makes validation of array results by additional array studies or by other methodologies (e.g., Northern blots) a dubious process. Statistical models based on inherent error properties, however, can account for differences among arrays and are easily validated. A differential judgment of expression based on a threshold significance probability of 0.05, for example, is the same across studies because it is based on both the difference between the signal intensities and on the random error associated with the difference. Accordingly, statistical methods provide a formal framework for (1) quality control, (2) establishing benchmarks against which the results of various studies can be compared, and (3) setting acceptable false positive and false negative error rates.

## Errors of Inference

FALSE POSITIVES
In order for two expression values to be considered reliably different from each other, their difference must exceed a threshold defined jointly by the random error associated with the difference and by a specified probability of concluding erroneously that the two values differ (false positive error rate).

Multiple discrete statistical tests, one for each transcript, are made in an array study. Therefore, there is an increased danger that we will accept positive findings that are actually due to chance.

To illustrate this point, let us adjust our significance criterion so that on any single test, we have less than a 5% chance of accepting a chance variation as significant. This is the familiar $p < 0.05$ criterion. If we perform this test on 10,000 spots, however, we can expect to find about 500 hits purely by chance. There are standard ways to correct for this tendency toward false positives. The basic principle is that the significance criterion is made more stringent, depending on the number of tests being performed.

One widely used correction for this problem is the Bonferroni procedure. In it, the nominal alpha level, say 0.05, is divided by the total number of tests to be performed. This "effective alpha" level is then used as the statistical significance threshold for each statistical test. In this way, we hold the probability of committing at least one false positive error somewhere in the entire set of analyses to the nominal alpha level of 0.05.

Other false-positive control procedures are less conservative than the Bonferroni procedure. A good example is the false discovery rate (FDR; Benjamini and Hochberg, 1995). The "false discovery rate" to be controlled by this procedure is the proportion of "hits" that we are willing to accept as erroneous. This criterion contrasts with the Bonferroni, which controls the probability of making at least one false positive error anywhere in the entire set of results. Corrections such as the FDR may fit the logic of some exploratory studies better than the Bonferroni does.

Note that both the Bonferroni and the FDR methods assume that genes do not exhibit correlated alterations in expression. Because groups of genes can fall into expression families, this assumption is not usually true. The consequence of this potential dependence is to overcorrect, making the correction more conservative than reality.

The use of false-positive error correction, although important, necessarily detracts further from sensitivity, with both parametric and nonparametric tests. With the Mann–Whitney test, for example, achieving a false-positive error rate of 0.01 requires a minimum of five replicates per gene, and the test will only be significant if all five replicates in one condition are ranked higher than those in the other condition. The correction is less severe with parametric tests, but still compounds the insensitivity of these tests with small sample sizes.

FALSE NEGATIVES

False negative errors are minimized by (1) increasing the number of replicates and (2) decreasing the random error across replicates by using more sensitive detection methods and experimental protocols. Both procedures reduce the random error associated with differences between averaged hybridization intensities. In the absence of a statistical framework, however, there is no way to quantify the false-negative error rate. Moreover, there is no way of even knowing if the false-negative error rate in a particular study is greater or less than the false-positive error rate. Accordingly, if effects of a particular magnitude are not found within a study, it is not known if this is because the effects did not exist or because the experiment was too insensitive to detect them. This additional shortcoming of nonstatistical approaches makes planning and assessing experiments a subjective and poorly defined process that varies from study to study.

In sum, many aspects of array analysis have been encumbered by nonstatistical approaches and by insensitive estimates of random error arising from small sample sizes. The resolution to this problem is discussed in a later section.

## Statistical Approaches

Statistical indices and tests have as their defining feature a decision as to whether it is likely that observed values reflect random error only or random error combined with treatment effect (i.e., "true difference"). The magnitude of random error that would be expected by chance is defined within the frequentist framework developed by Fisher (1925).

In this framework, probability is assessed by reference to distributions of repeated measurements of the same attribute or process. Differences between experimental conditions are assessed relative to random variation within conditions. Methods for estimating these terms depend on the experimental design. In all cases, however, if the between variation exceeds the within variation by the predefined alpha level (false positive error rate), the observed differences are considered statistically significant.

### Signal-to-Noise Methods

"Signal-to-noise" methods attempt to discriminate differentially expressed genes (signal) relative to the large number of genes that do not show differences in expression (noise). These methods are based on distribution properties of the array data, and their advocates cite the advantage that they do not require replicate measurements of any type.

For example, Chen et al. (1997) estimate the statistical significance of changes in expression from the distribution of non-replicated differential ratios as expected under the null hypothesis. The method assumes a constant random error for all raw score ratios, as indexed by the coefficient of variation. Thus, the CV of the expression values allows predictions about how those values are distributed, and values that deviate from the expected distribution are taken as meaningful.

In practice, the CV is estimated from a set of nonreplicated reference genes which (theoretically) are unrelated to the experimental condition. The CV estimate taken from these genes is used to generate the sampling distribution of the ratios under the null hypothesis. That is, the method derives what the distribution of ratios would be if all of the spots showed "chance" differences in expression values across conditions. Based on this derivation of random noise, thresholds are established for statistically reliable ratios. Newton et al. (2000) have presented a modification of the approach within a Bayesian framework.

Signal-to-noise approaches are attractive in that they promise objective assessments of differential expression in nonreplicated two-color arrays. They are most useful when a large number of observations must be made, but material costs are high. As costs per spot decrease, however, the advantages of obtaining duplicate or triplicate measurements (outlier detection, more reliable measurements) may outweigh the cost savings from the use of non-replicated data.

A limitation of some signal-to-noise methods is that they were designed for two-color fluorescent applications. It is unclear how applicable these methods are to other array paradigms (e.g., radio-isotopic, single-color fluorescence). An additional concern is that the methods assume normally distributed error on the raw scale. It is not clear how robust the methods are with respect to violation of the normality assumption. This is a potentially important consideration in light of the emerging consensus that random error for array applications is lognormal.

It is also assumed that all measured values are unbiased and reliable estimates of the "true" spot intensity. That is, it is assumed that none of the spot intensities are outliers that should be excluded from analysis. Indeed, outlier detection in the conventional sense is not possible with this approach. Therefore, the methods are completely dependent upon pixel-based outlier removal within the image quantification software.

A somewhat different approach, using similar principles, has been developed for single-condition radioisotopic arrays (Piétu et al., 1996). These authors observed that a histogram of spot intensities in their data presented a bimodal distribution, and that the distribution of the low signal values appeared to follow a Gaussian distribution dominated by random error. Accordingly, they fitted the distribution of these low-intensity values to a Gaussian curve and used a threshold of 1.96 standard deviations above the mean of the curve to distinguish nonsignal noise intensities (smaller than the threshold) from signals (larger than the threshold). The method is appropriate for single-condition studies only because it does not readily allow comparisons across conditions. Also, the method tends to be insensitive in that the false negative error rate can be high. This tendency is most pronounced when there is a greater degree of overlap between the low-signal Gaussian curve and the distribution of high signal values.

Yet another approach is based on the exploratory statistical technique of analyzing principal components (Hilsenbeck et al., 1999). Principal components analysis is a method for grouping correlated measurements into a smaller number of uncorrelated variables. In the example cited, radioisotopic data were used to isolate genes based on patterns of expression and not on error estimates per se. The authors extracted three components from the data. Based on their pattern of expression, individual genes were classified as being differentially expressed or not. The authors discuss simulations that lend support to their results and advocate their method for single-measurement studies. They conclude that the method is a cost-effective way to screen genes for more intensive follow-up. Wittes and Friedman (1999) have criticized the approach, however, arguing that the only way to minimize the likely large number of false positives generated by the method is to obtain replicates. Moreover, false-negative error control is not possible with the method.

### Proxy Methods

Proxy methods attempt to retain the classical frequentist paradigm of obtaining random error estimates from replicated measurements, but without requiring replicates for each spot in the array. Estimates are obtained from proxies that are not expected to exhibit systematic variation linked to the experimental conditions. As with systematic error correction and outlier detection, the two main sources for proxy estimates of random error are background on the digitized image and reference genes (Duggan et al., 1999; Ermolaeva et al., 1998).

DeRisi et al. (1997), for example, used variance thresholds based on background variation. Ratio intensities were considered significant if they exceeded 2.5 times the standard deviation of the background pixels. Schena et al. (1996) examined only those ratios whose difference across duplicate measurements was less than half of the average of the duplicate ratios. In this way, ratios that demonstrated large variation across duplicate measurements were excluded from further analysis. Of the remaining values, only those that showed greater than twofold changes were considered significant. By considering the distance between replicate values, Schena et al. used an informal fold-change approach that also acknowledged random error.

Proxy methods suffer because the estimate of measurement error is not obtained directly from the data of interest. The error operating on the proxy values may or may not coincide with the data error, especially as the data points deviate from the intensity values of the proxies.

A more flexible approach taken with double-fluorescent data (Hughes et al., 2000) uses multiple estimates of random error, including those from single measurements, proxies, and replicates, as available. For example, the authors describe a single-array (no replicates) random-error model that differs from the model proposed by Chen et al. (1997) in part because it includes an estimate of error that is due to deficiencies in background correction. The single-error estimate obtained for the entire array is combined with error estimates obtained from replicates and from same vs. same control experiments when available. The error model weights the different estimates differentially, depending on the quality of information available from each source.

Although the method requires a relatively large number of replicated control experiments to be optimal, it represents the first systematic attempt to combine error estimates from numerous extraneous factors. As these sources of error come under better experimental control, the model's complexity will most likely be reduced.

### Pooled Error Methods

The method that we propose for estimating random error is based on a simple concept. While there may be few replicates for each specific gene, there are large numbers of genes per array. Each gene represents an individual experiment, and an array, then, presents a large number of small sample experiments tested under the same conditions. Given this, it should be possible to pool the random error estimates across all genes. In retrospect, this is an obvious approach. The difficulty lies in validating the underlying assumption that the global estimate of random error is an accurate estimate for the discrete-sample error terms.

For this assumption to be true, these discrete error terms must all belong to the same population. To evaluate this hypothesis, we have done two things. We have conducted simulation studies in which the population variance is known, and then recovered that population variance from the pooling process. We have also examined how the pooled error method performs with real array data. An example of real-world validation is presented later.

We have developed two variants of the pooled error method, which we refer to as "common error" and "fitted," to estimate the random error associated with each transcript. Unlike the methods discussed earlier, our pooled error methods estimate random error from the entire array and can function with as few as two replicates. Because our random error estimates are based on large samples, they provide more accurate (through better outlier removal) and more precise estimates than other methods. With these accurate error estimates in hand, classical statistical techniques can be applied to array analyses. Although our methods were initially validated with printed arrays, they appear to be equally appropriate to microfabricated arrays and to other applications in which there are large numbers of small-sample experiments.

The common error method simply pools the error estimates obtained for each gene in each condition, and is best used when standard deviations are unrelated to intensity. The fitted method estimates random error using a robust nonparametric spline fit (He and Shi, 1998; Shi, 1995). The fitted method pools error estimates locally, based on the curve fit and has the advantage that it applies when data exhibit a relation between signal intensity and standard deviation.

## An Example of an Inferential Analysis

We illustrate the principles of our approach by offering a reanalysis of a public data set. While varying data sets (e.g., fluorescent vs. radioisotopic) offer different challenges, the selected set (Tanaka et al., 2000, http://lgsun.grc.nia.nih.gov/array/) is representative of many common problems in array analysis. These radioisotopic data compare gene expression across mouse embryonic and placental tissues. There are three replicates in each condition, yielding a total of six columns of data values, one row for each of the 15,264 genes. We describe each step in the analysis procedure without detailing the tools used to accomplish that step.

### Necessary Preliminaries: Cleaning Up the Data

The raw data were inspected to determine whether the range of values was sensible. This dataset presents evidence of clipping (floor) effects. For each of the arrays, there is a single lowest expression value that appears at high frequency. For example, the first replicate set for the embryonic tissue had 3292 genes with an intensity value (in arbitrary units of the quantification software) of 1.02. This suggests that the detector offset is set to yield this value in a no-signal condition. Clipped values (and saturated values) represent errors of the image acquisition process (rather than of the arrays) and must be excluded so that they do not bias subsequent statistical analysis.

Plotting the standard deviation vs. the mean for all of the genes (figure 4.2) revealed a positive relationship between the standard deviations and their respective condition means. A log transformation of the data values is required to reduce or remove this relationship between the standard deviation and the mean. Removing such a relationship is important, both to meet the assumptions of the upcoming statistical tests and to make results comparable across intensities.

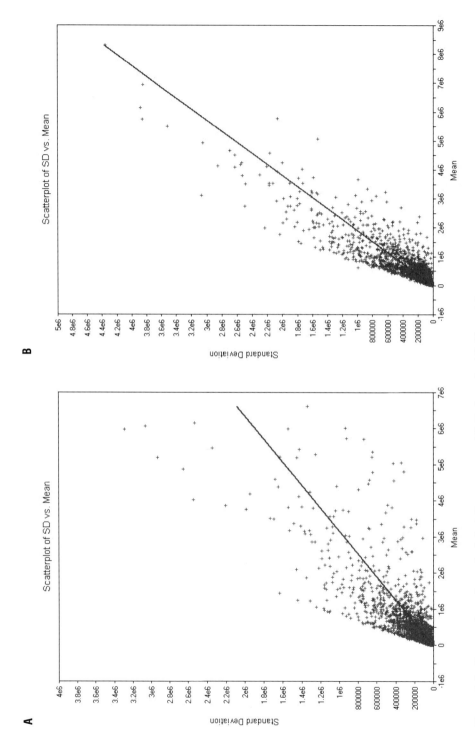

**Figure 4.2** Scatter plots of standard deviation vs. mean. (*A*) Embryonic. (*B*) Placental.

## Dependent vs. Independent Tests

Dual-color microarrays tend to present dependent data because targets from two conditions hybridize to the same probe, causing dependence between the measurements. With independent data, by contrast, there is no systematic relationship (correlation) between replicates in one condition and replicates in another. Different statistical tests are applicable in the two circumstances. In the present case, the six replicate sets were obtained from discrete membranes. Therefore, procedures appropriate for independent samples were used during outlier detection and in subsequent tests.

## Common Error or Fitted

Figure 4.3 (see also plate 4) shows graphs of standard deviations across the range of replicate means for the logged data. Ideally, the log transform would have removed any relationship between mean and standard deviation. With the present data, this is not true for the full range. Signal intensities of approximately 4 and above show no relationship of mean to standard deviation. Below 4, however, there is a pronounced negative relationship between mean and standard deviation. This pattern is often seen with radioisotopic data and probably reflects a property of the phosphor imaging technology used to visualize the array. Storage phosphor plates (unlike film) tend to exhibit proportionately higher noise at low signal intensities (Duggan et al., 1999).

Given the relationship observed between signal intensity and standard deviation, the common error method would not be appropriate. Therefore the fitted method was used, in which a nonparametric spline function was approximated to each of the scatter plots. From the spline fit, an estimate of the error for each level of mean signal intensity was derived. This method provides the common error solution for the range for which it is appropriate (4 and above), while accommodating increasing error estimates in the range below 4.

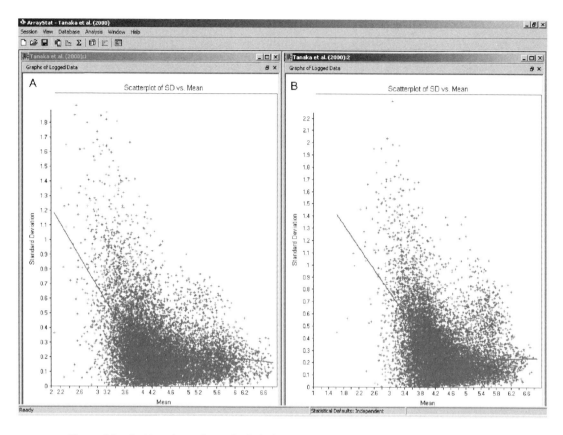

**Figure 4.3** Scatter plots of standard deviation vs. mean: logged values. (*A*) Embryonic. (*B*) Placental. See plate 4 for color version.

Some datasets (a small minority) neither show the common error property (horizontal best-fit line across the whole range of signal intensities), nor yield any plausible fitted curve. This circumstance would occur if there were a nonstraightforward relationship between mean and standard deviation. The pooled error technique is not appropriate for such data, and it may be more appropriate to use conventional statistical tests that estimate error from the data for that gene alone. As we will see, having to fall back on this "small sample" approach entails considerable drawbacks.

## Normalization and Outliers

Thus far, we have determined that certain values must be treated as missing, that the data need to be log transformed, and that a curve fit approach can be used to estimate error for the upcoming statistical tests. The next two issues to deal with are normalization across replicates within the same experimental condition (what we call "offset correction") and detection of outliers.

We distinguish between two types of normalization. In the first instance, we wish to correct for systematic error across replicates of the same experimental condition (tissue, etc.). We call this within-condition normalization "offset correction." In the second instance, we wish to correct for systematic error across conditions (between-condition normalization). In each case, it is best to center the corrected values rather than bring the values to a mean of 1 (or to a mean of 0 in log space).

To understand the distinction between the two normalization procedures, consider the following. In the case of arrays within any particular condition, the arrays are exact replicates. Therefore, differences in observed mean array intensities are most likely due to systematic error. In the absence of other information, the mean of all the arrays is the best estimate of the true mean. Hence, the values within the arrays are adjusted to bring the mean of each array to the overall mean of all the arrays. That is, the values are "centered."

In the case of arrays across different conditions, matters are more complicated; a difference in average array intensities may be due to systematic error, a condition effect, or some combination of the two. Between-condition normalization must address this potential for an overall condition effect. If a large proportion of genes are truly differentially expressed, for example, correcting for systematic error in the usual way removes some of the condition effect for the genes that are differentially expressed and potentially creates differences between genes that are not truly different. Normalizing within and between conditions separately has the added advantage of allowing us to apply different normalization methods as appropriate (e.g., normalize to the mean for within-condition normalization, and normalize to reference values for between-condition normalization).

The presence of outliers further complicates normalization. In a sense, it is a chicken-and-egg problem. We want to remove systematic error before selecting outliers, but we want to remove outliers prior to calculating systematic error. Therefore, we conduct offset correction and outlier detection in an iterative fashion. That is, after an initial offset correction of the data, a first pass is made to identify outliers. Then, omitting those outliers, the offset correction of the surviving observations is recomputed. Next, a second pass is made to identify additional outliers, and so forth. When no further outliers are found (using predefined criteria), all surviving observations are offset corrected for the last time.

The effect of this iterative outlier detection procedure is shown in figure 4.4. Panels A and B depict characteristics of the logged data for placental tissue before the procedure, and panels C and D show the corresponding characteristics afterward. In the panels at the top (A and C), we have histograms of residuals, which are useful for showing the relative frequency of extreme values. Each residual is a data value minus the mean for that gene, weighted by a function of sample size and standardized by the error estimate to give approximately unit variance in the resulting residuals.

Note that in panel A, we have what appears to be a reasonably Gaussian distribution, but it is contaminated on both sides (here, especially the low side) by extreme values. In the corresponding histogram of residuals after the procedure, shown in panel C, these outliers have been eliminated. In addition, we have the expected normal distribution with unit variance, with values falling in the range of $-3$ to $+3$ (although the tails are slightly heavy).

The presence or absence of outliers is more readily apparent in the associated quantile-quantile (Q-Q) plots, shown as panels B and D. A Q-Q plot displays the observed standardized residual values (x-axis) against the expected values for a perfect Gaussian distribution (y-axis). If all of the residuals were perfectly normally

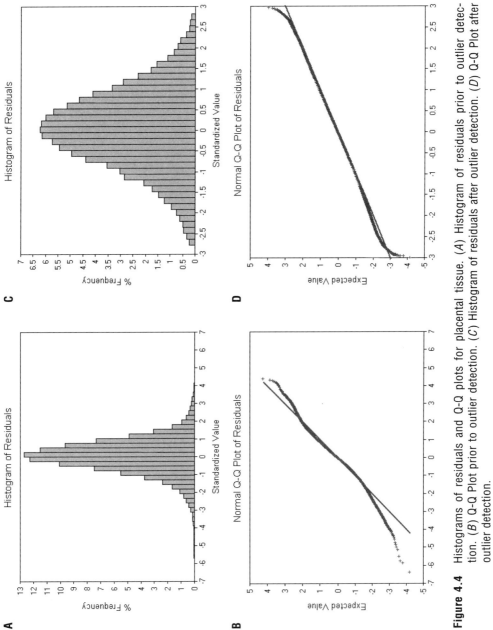

**Figure 4.4** Histograms of residuals and Q-Q plots for placental tissue. (*A*) Histogram of residuals prior to outlier detection. (*B*) Q-Q Plot prior to outlier detection. (*C*) Histogram of residuals after outlier detection. (*D*) Q-Q Plot after outlier detection.

distributed, the observed values would fall exactly along the solid diagonal line of expected values. In panel B, we see outliers at both ends of the solid line. These are eliminated in the corresponding panel (D) after outlier detection and offset correction have been performed. The process and results for embryonic tissue are virtually the same.

At this point, the raw data have been log transformed to make them more amenable to statistical analysis; systematic error within each condition has been adjusted out by normalization; and clipped values and outliers have been removed. For the placental tissue, 10,253 of the 45,792 original observations (22.4%) were excluded owing to clipping, and 815 further observations (1.8%) were eliminated as outliers, for a total of 11,068 (24.2%) excluded values. The numbers for the embryonic tissue data are 7,126 (15.6%) missing and 929 (2.0%) outliers, for a total of 8,055 (17.6%) excluded values. Note that although the proportion of observations detected as outliers is small, the sheer number is quite large. Such cleaning of data has an important and widespread impact on subsequent statistical tests.

### Normalizing across Conditions

For cross-condition normalization, normalizing "by mean" uses a centering process that brings the average difference between conditions, computed across all the genes, to 0. As mentioned earlier, unless the number of differentially expressed genes is small, the adjustment can remove real effects to some degree; it can also separate the means of unexpressed genes in a direction opposite to the genuine effects obtained with other genes in the array.

There are alternative ways to normalize that help overcome these problems. For example, we could use reference genes, predesignated as unlikely to be differentially expressed, and adjust the data so that the mean difference between conditions for these reference genes is 0. Another possibility is iterative normalization by mean, which involves removing differentially expressed genes in successive steps, recalculating the normalization reference between each step.

Nonetheless, we applied normalization by mean without iteration to the present dataset because we expected that the vast majority of genes would not be differentially expressed. It is therefore reasonable to assume that any difference in the overall means for the two conditions reflects systematic error (rather than overall differences between the tissues) and should be adjusted out.

### Statistical Tests

Because our random error estimate based on the curve fit is precise, we are justified in using $z$-tests rather than the more conventional $t$-tests. A $z$-test uses the standard normal distribution for establishing significance thresholds, which makes it more sensitive to small effects, especially when sample sizes are small.

With the present dataset, 12,682 genes could be submitted for statistical tests. The Bonferroni-corrected "effective alpha" is 0.0000039426 (0.05/12,682), producing 76 differentially expressed genes (0.5% of the entire set of genes), all of which are in the direction of placental tissue exceeding embryonic tissue. Using the FDR alpha correction procedure (FDR = 0.05), we found 269 differentially expressed genes (1.8%), of which 242 showed greater expression for placental tissue and 27 showed the reverse. The difference in number of differentially expressed genes found with the two procedures illustrates that selection of an appropriate type of false-positive error correction is important.

### Conclusion

Using simple $t$-tests on the raw data without log transform, uncorrected for outliers or for false-positive error due to multiple tests, Tanaka et al. report 720 positives in their data. Given their alpha level of 0.05, this number is about the proportion that could be expected from chance. Tanaka et al. do report Northern blot confirmation for five positive and five negative findings. Our statistical analysis (Bonferroni and FDR) concurred with the results of the Northerns for eight of the genes (four placenta positives and four genes not differentially expressed), but overall it suggests a high false-positive error rate. We rejected the ninth gene, which the Northern blot identified as being embryonic specific, because of clipped values for all of the placental replicates. We were unable to locate the tenth gene because its label differed from place to place in the report by Tanaka et al.

Finally, it is interesting to compare the results using pooled error methods with the results obtained with more conventional procedures: individual $t$-tests on each gene with log transformation, outlier removal, and alpha error correction. Using either the FDR or the Bonferroni procedure, the resulting 12,682 $t$-tests failed to find even a single "hit."

Uncorrected $t$-tests would appear to do "better"; with no alpha correction, there are 1083 hits (7.1% of all the genes). The momentary elation of finding so many apparent results should, however, be tempered by the realization that most are likely to be false-positive errors. There is no way of knowing a priori which of these "significantly" expressed genes are the false positives.

We have described a novel process for conducting inferential analyses of genome arrays with high sensitivity while minimizing false positive errors. The application of this process to large bodies of data is straightforward and has been incorporated into a commercially available software package. As more tools for statistical analysis become available to array researchers, we expect to see rapid formalization and standardization of analytical methods. This will greatly ease the application of a powerful technology to questions in neuroscience.

## References

Bartosiewicz M, Trounstine M, Barker D, Johnston R, and Buckpitt A (2000). Development of a toxicological gene array and quantitative assessment of this technology. *Arch Biochem Biophys* 376: 66–73.

Bassett DE, Eisen MB, and Boguski MS (1999). Gene expression informatics: It's all in your mine. *Nat Genet* 21: 51–5.

Benjamini Y and Hochberg Y (1995). Controlling the false discovery rate: A practical and powerful approach to multiple testing. *J Roy Statistical Soc Ser B, Methodological* 57: 289–300.

Brown PO and Botstein D (1999). Exploring the new world of the genome with DNA microarrays. *Nat Genet* 21: 33–7.

Chen Y, Dougherty ER, and Bittner ML (1997). Ratio-based decisions and the quantitative analysis of cDNA microarray images. *J Biomedical Optics* 2: 364–74.

Claverie JM (1999). Computational methods for the identification of differential and coordinated gene expression. *Human Mol Genet* 8: 1821–32.

Cole KA, Krizman DB, and Emmert-Buck MR (1999). The genetics of cancer—a 3D model. *Nat Genet* 21: 38–41.

DeRisi JL, Iyer VR, and Brown PO (1997). Exploring the metabolic and genetic control of gene expression on a genomic scale. *Science* 278: 680–6.

Duggan DJ, Bittner M, Chen YD, Meltzer P, and Trent JM (1999). Expression profiling using cDNA microarrays. *Nat Genet* 21: 10–14.

Eickhoff B, Korn B, Schick M, Poustka A, and van der Bosch J (1999). Normalization of array hybridization experiments in differential gene expression analysis. *Nucleic Acids Res Meth* 27: 22–4.

Ermolaeva O, Rastogi M, Pruitt KD, Schuker GD, Bittner ML, Chen Y, Simon R, Meltzer P, Trent JM, and Boguski MS (1998). Data management and analysis for gene expression arrays. *Nat Genet* 20: 19–23.

Fisher RA (1925). *Statistical Methods for Research Workers.* Oliver and Boyd, Edinburgh.

Geiss GK, Bumgarner RE, An MC, Agy MB, Van't Wout AB, Hammersmark E, Carter VS, Upchurch D, Mullins JI, and Katze MG (2000). Large-scale monitoring of host cell gene expression during HIV-1 infection using cDNA microarrays. *Virology* 266: 8–16.

Goodman L (1999). Hypothesis-limited research. *Genome Res* 9: 673–4.

He X and Shi P (1998). Monotone *B*-spline smoothing. *J Am Statistical Assoc* 93: 643–50.

Hilsenbeck SG, Friedrichs WE, Schiff R, O'Connell P, Hansen RK, Osborne CK, and Fuqua SAW (1999). Statistical analysis of array expression data as applied to the problem of tamoxifen resistance. *J Nat Cancer Inst* 91: 453–9.

Hughes TR, Marton MJ, Jones AR, Roberts CJ, Stoughton R, Armour CD, Bennett HA, Coffey E, et al. (2000). Functional discovery via a compendium of expression profiles. *Cell* 102: 109–26.

Lander ES (1999). Array of hope. *Nat Genet* 21: 3–4.

Lee MLT, Kuo FC, Whitmore GA, and Sklar J (2000). Importance of replication in microarray gene expression studies: Statistical methods and evidence from repetitive cDNA hybridizations. *Proc Nat Acad Sci USA* 97: 9834–9.

Newton MA, Kendziorski CM, Richmond CS, Blattner FR, and Tsui KW (2001). On differential variability of expression ratios: Improving statistical inference about gene expression changes from microarray data. *Journal of Computational Biology* 8: 37–52.

Perret E, Ferrán EA, Marinx O, Liauzun P, Dumont X, Fournier J, Kaghad M, Ferrara P, and Caput D (1998). Improved differential screening approach to analyse transcriptional variations in organized cDNA libraries. *Gene* 208: 103–15.

Piétu G, Alibert O, Guichard V, Lamy B, Bois F, Leroy E, Mariage-Samson R, Houlgatte R, Soularue P, and Auffray C (1996). Novel gene transcripts preferentially expressed in human muscles revealed by quantitative hybridization of a high density cDNA array. *Genome Res* 6: 492–503.

Schena M, Shalon D, Heller R, Chai A, Brown PO, and Davis RW (1996). Parallel human genome analysis: Microarray-based expression monitoring of 1000 genes. *Proc Nat Acad Sci USA* 93: 10614–19.

Shalon D, Smith SJ, and Brown PO (1996). A DNA microarray system for analyzing complex DNA samples using two-color fluorescent probe hybridization. *Genome Res* 6: 639–45.

Sherlock G (2000). Analysis of large-scale gene expression data. *Curr Opinion Immunol* 12: 201–5.

Shi P (1995). Some new results of *M*-type regression spline estimators in a partial linear model. *Kexue Tongbao* (China) 39: 189–92.

Staudt LM (2000). Immunological techniques—the expression of the genome during immune responses—Editorial Overview. *Curr Opinion Immunol* 12: 199–200.

Tanaka T, Jaradat S, Lim M, Kargul G, Wang X, Grahovac M, Pantano S, Sano Y, Piao Y, Nagaraja R, Doi H, Wood WH, Becker K, and Ko M (2000). Genome-wide expression profiling of mid-gestation placenta and embryo using a 15,000 mouse developmental cDNA microarray. *Proc Natl Acad Sci USA* 97: 9127–32.

Wittes J and Friedman HP (1999). Searching for evidence of altered gene expression: A comment on statistical analysis of microarray data. *J Natl Cancer Inst* 91: 400–1.

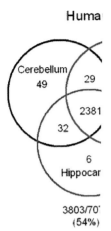

Huma

Cerebellum 49 | 29

2381

32

6
Hippocar

3803/70
(54%)

**Plate 5** Of mouse an
set of adult human ar
fied as "present" in a
sify genes as clearly r
levels below the thres
scored as present in
centage of genes are
may be because only
from the smaller mou

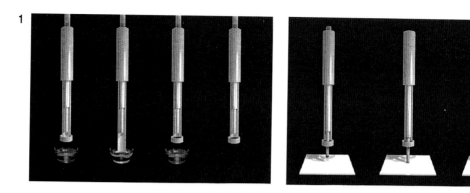

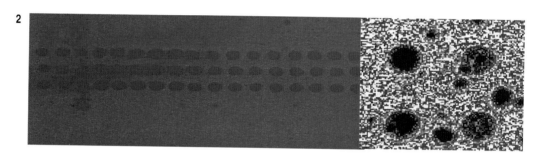

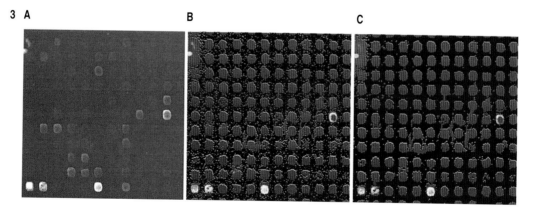

**Plate 1** Pin-and-Ring system from Affymetrix (formerly Genetic Microsystems). See chapter 1.
**Plate 2** Contamination in microarray images may be seen in both the background and inside the spots. See chapter 3.
**Plate 3** Comparison between median filtering (B) and combined local statistics adaptive filtering (C) as applied to an example microarray image (A). See chapter 3.

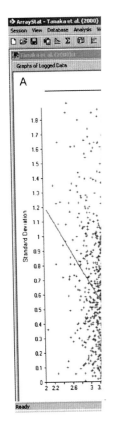

**Plate 4** Scatter p

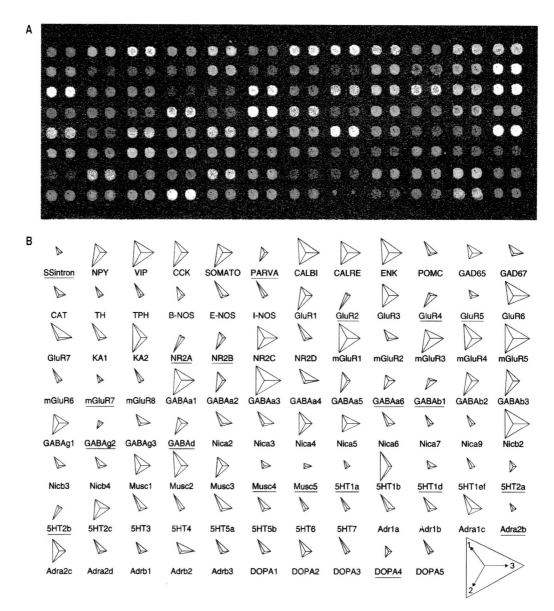

**Plate 7** (A) Hybridization to the Neurochip of multiplex PCR products obtained from cDNA quantities corresponding to a one-cell content. The spectrum of colors corresponds to the level of fluorescent signal: from black-blue to white for increasing intensities. (B) Star plot for analyzing multiplex PCR for amplifying 94 genes in one tube. Axis 1, multiplex PCR from DNA targets; axis 2, agarose RT-PCR; axis 3, multiplex PCR from cDNA corresponding to (A). See chapter 9.

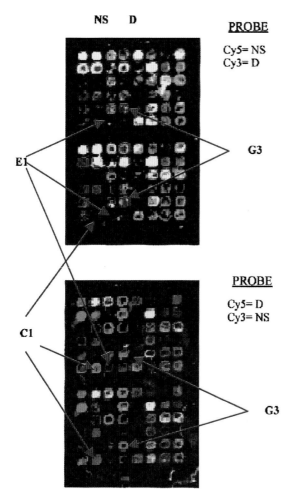

NS    D

PROBE

Cy5= NS
Cy3= D

G3

E1

PROBE

Cy5= D
Cy3= NS

C1

G3

**Plate 8** Magnified microarray quadrants. Magnified false color images of a pilot microarray of RDA round 2 subtraction products. Clones from the NS-D direction are arrayed in the first four columns on the left side of the array under NS, and those from the D-NS direction are arrayed in columns 5–6 on the right under D. Both arrays shown are duplicates of each other, with the labeling dyes switched to indicate that the differential labeling represents differential hybridization and is not an artifact of the probe label. See chapter 10.

# 5 cDNA Array Strategies and Alternative Approaches in Neuroscience: Focus on Radioactive Probes

*Kevin G. Becker, Tanya Barrett, and Laurie W. Whitney*

The large-scale expressed sequence tag (EST) sequencing projects have produced over one million cDNA clones representing over 65,000 unique cDNA clusters. This may represent a majority of all human genes. Recently, estimates of the number of unique human genes have been revised from more than 100,000 to fewer than 50,000 (Hattori et al., 2000; Dunham et al., 1999; Ewing and Green, 2000). These cDNA collections have allowed the assembly and use of cDNA arrays for hybridization-based profiling of gene expression.

cDNA arrays allow the parallel analysis of gene expression patterns in thousands of genes simultaneously under a similar set of experimental conditions, thus making the data highly comparable (Schena et al., 1995; Duggan et al., 1999). Quite often the goal of expression profiling is to begin to identify complex regulatory networks underlying developmental processes and disease states. In other cases, arrays are used as a primary screen leading to downstream molecular characterization and validation of individual gene candidates.

This cDNA library hybridization approach is simply an extension of the differential cDNA library screening first done in 1983 (Sargent and Dawid, 1983). Important differences from earlier de novo cDNA screening efforts of the 1980s and early 1990s include:

1. Increased information content about the cDNA clones, such as the partial or full-length cDNA sequence, chromosomal map position, tissue distribution, and in some cases functional inferences caused by sequence homology
2. The use of fluorescent labeling techniques and glass substrates
3. Improved high-throughput technical approaches such as 96- or 384-well plasmid preparations and PCR techniques
4. Improved software for data archiving and analysis.

There are a number of alternatives available in expression arrays, for example, oligonucleotide chips and cDNA arrays, each with associated advantages and disadvantages. Some important aspects in choosing an array approach are technical whereas others are practical. The use of expression arrays for neuroscience applications presents unique problems. Often, use and analysis of cDNA arrays from complex brain tissue or small regions of tissue is more difficult than for those from cell lines or pure tissue sources. The type of array approach used should be taken into account when planning a particular screening effort or experimental protocol.

## cDNA Array Collections

Large sequenced human, mouse, and rat cDNA collections are available for purchase from a number of commercial sources, including Invitrogen, Inc.; Incyte, Inc.; and the American Type Culture Collection, among others. These clone sets usually contain from 5000 to 20,000 cDNA clones stored as plasmid-containing bacterial colonies. All the clone inserts can be PCR amplified with standard sets of PCR primers.

The quality and reproducibility of array data are obviously highly dependent on the quality of the underlying clones used to construct the arrays. Some problems with cDNA array collections until recently have included incorrect sequence identification, multiple clones per well, and bacteriophage T1 contamination of the clone cultures. Recent versions of the publicly available cDNA collections have been colony purified, sequenced, and transformed in T1-resistant bacteria. These potential problems should be taken into account when choosing commercially available clone sources. For example, Invitrogen, Inc. currently has clone sets with these quality controls, but other commercial clone sets derived from IMAGE Consortium cDNA clones may not have such quality controls incorporated.

Many laboratories also have made private collections of empirically derived clones resulting from EST sequencing projects, differential display, or other cDNA screening efforts. For example, Tanaka and colleagues (2000) have assembled a nonredundant collection of 15,264 unique cDNAs derived from early murine developmental cDNA libraries. This collection has been arrayed to study genome-wide murine embryonic development. In addition, in chapter 10 Geschwind and Nelson describe how cDNA subtractions may also provide a useful source of empirically derived libraries for gene expression studies.

Similarly, logically derived clones are assembled into collections of functionally related clones (signal transduction, apoptosis, etc.) for specific applications. The choice of a particular cDNA clone collection is independent of the array format used. PCR products from any clone source can be spotted equivalently on glass or filter supports (see also chapter 6).

The National Institute on Aging (NIA) Neuroarray is an example of a logically derived set of cDNA clones for neural applications (Barrett et al., 2001, Vawter et al., 2001). This is a collection of 1152 human cDNAs rearrayed from IMAGE Consortium human cDNAs that code for genes expressed in human neural tissues. A summary of gene categories with selected examples of elements found in the NIA Neuroarray is shown in table 5.1. This array is being used for studies in neurodegeneration, drug toxicity, and neurodevelopment, among other applications. In many experimental situations it is more practical to use smaller, logically defined, focused sets of cDNAs rather than randomly chosen large arrays. High cost, limiting amounts of RNA, or large sample numbers often make the screening of large arrays (10–20,000 cDNAs) impractical.

**Array Formats**

There are two basic formats of arrayed cDNA collections: (1) cDNAs attached to glass microscope slides (Schena et al., 1995; DeRisi et al., 1996) or (2) cDNAs attached to nylon membranes (Tanaka et al., 2000; Barrett et al., 2001). Oligonucleotide-based chips (Lipshutz et al., 1999) are not discussed here. A more recent

**Table 5.1** Summary of genes found in the National Institute on Aging Neuroarray

| | UNIGENE NUMBER |
|---|---|
| *Cell adhesion molecules* | |
| Selectin E (endothelial adhesion molecule 1) | Hs.89546 |
| Selectin L (lymphocyte adhesion molecule 1) | Hs.82848 |
| Intercellular adhesion molecule 1 (CD54) | Hs.168383 |
| Neural cell adhesion molecule | Hs.210863 |
| Opioid-binding cell adhesion molecule | Hs.99902 |
| *Receptors* | |
| Adrenergic beta-2-receptor | Hs.2551 |
| Cannabinoid receptor 1 | Hs.75110 |
| Cholinergic receptor nicotinic epsilon | Hs.112028 |
| Corticotropin releasing factor receptor 1 | Hs.79117 |
| Epidermal growth factor receptor | Hs.77432 |
| *Transporters* | |
| Neurotransmitter transporter, noradrenalin | Hs.78036 |
| Neurotransmitter transporter, GABA | Hs.2682 |
| Axonal transporter of synaptic vesicles | Hs.75096 |
| Glutamate transporter | Hs.75379 |
| Glucose transporter, brain | Hs.7594 |
| *Growth factors* | |
| Brain-derived neurotrophic factor | Hs.56023 |
| Leukemia inhibitory factor | Hs.2250 |
| Nerve growth factor beta | Hs.2561 |
| Platelet-derived growth factor beta | Hs.1976 |
| Transforming growth factor beta 2 | Hs.169300 |
| *Channels* | |
| Potassium voltage-gated channel | Hs.172471 |
| Calcium channel, voltage-dependent | Hs.23838 |
| Chloride intracellular channel 1 | Hs.74276 |
| Potassium inwardly rectifying channel | Hs.17287 |
| Voltage-dependent anion channel form 3 | Hs.7381 |
| Total human cDNAs arrayed in duplicate | 1152 |

intermediate version of cDNA support is through nitrocellulose-coated glass slides (Grace Bio-Labs, Inc.) or nylon-coated glass slides (Schleicher & Schuell, Inc.). These filter-coated glass slides fit into most DNA array spotting machines and provide a flat surface for spotting and a convenient way to process and store small filter arrays. Membrane-coated slides are relatively new and have not been tested rigorously under varied experimental conditions. For protocols on cDNA labeling of RNA, membrane hybridization, washing, exposure, and stripping, see the protocols at the end of this chapter.

### Glass Slides using Fluorescent Probes

cDNA arrays using glass microscope slides are generally custom made in academic centers (Schena et al., 1995; DeRisi et al., 1996; Whitney et al., 1999), although some commercial sources are becoming available (e.g., Perkin Elmer Life Sciences [formerly NEN Life Sciences], Corning Inc., BD Biosciences). The purified cDNA PCR products are robotically attached to the surface of the glass either through poly-L-lysine or silane surface coating. Purified PCR products are spotted in high density at approximately 100–400 µm spacing, center to center. This allows approximately 5–15,000 spots per standard 1 × 3-inch glass microscope slide. The positive signals from these targets using fluorescent probes have clearly defined edges and easily distinguishable signals. (In this chapter, the terms *probe* and *target* are used as they are commonly used in molecular biology. Probe refers to the labeled unknown pool of cDNA or RNA while target(s) refers to the known cDNA spot(s) attached to a solid support.)

Hybridization on the glass surface is generally performed as a two-color comparative hybridization under a cover slip in a low volume of hybridization solution (10–100 µl), thereby concentrating the probe. Although glass slides are used for two probes simultaneously, they are single-use slides and cannot be stripped and reused. When used with fluorescently labeled probes, glass-based arrays require custom-built or, more recently, commercially available fluorescent scanners and dedicated software.

### Membrane or Filter-Based Arrays

The use of membrane-based solution hybridization is a well-established approach for differential expression studies (Sargent and Dawid, 1983). Membrane-based microarrays are generally used with [33]P-dCTP or [33]P-dATP radiolabeled probes (Zhao et al., 1995; Pietu et al., 1996; Bertucci et al., 1999) although colorimetric reporter systems have been used (Chen et al., 1998).[1] The spot-to-spot spacing for commercial filter arrays or custom filter arrays is generally greater than approximately 500 μm because of bleeding over of adjacent strong radioactive spots.

The use of radioactive probes inhibits close cDNA spot packing. This allows approximately 2000–3000 spots to be placed on a standard $25 \times 75$-mm microscope slide. These spots can be easily resolved at 50 μm on a phosphoimaging system, such as the STORM phosphoimager from Amersham Biosciences. Exposure times are generally from 1 to 3 days. Membrane arrays can be stripped and reused at least three to five times and in this respect have an advantage over glass arrays, which are currently not reusable.

The NIA Neuroarray (Barrett et al., 2001) is an example of a membrane cDNA array. This is a collection of 1152 logically determined neural cDNAs. Figure 5.1 shows cDNAs arrayed in duplicate on nylon membranes (Schleicher & Schuell Supercharge+). This is printed at 665-μm spot-to-spot spacing, giving 2304 total spots for approximately $20 \times 70$ mm. These minimembrane arrays are hybridized in 4 ml of hybridization solution in disposable 50-ml centrifuge tubes overnight at $50\,^{\circ}$C.

### Glass Slides using Radioactive Probes

Glass slides have also been used with more traditional [33]P-dCTP labeled probes, allowing the use of smaller tissue samples (Whitney

A                                      B

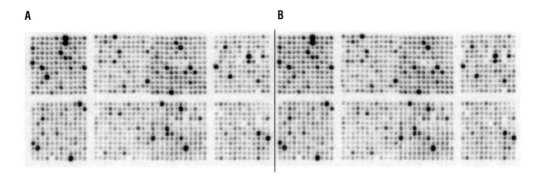

**Figure 5.1**  National Institute on Aging Neuroarray.

et al., 1999; Whitney and Becker, 2001). The use of $^{33}$P-dCTP-labeled probes on glass slides is largely dependent on spot density. Using glass slides with $^{33}$P-labeled probes allows the use of very small hybridization volumes (10–100 µl). This allows the use of probes with high specific activity ($> 10^9$ cpm/ml) and in turn requires smaller quantities of tissue and total RNA (50–100 mg of tissue or 50 ng to 5 µg total RNA) per experiment. When used with $^{33}$P-dCTP-labeled probes, glass and filter arrays can generally be used with 1–10 µg of total RNA. This is quite often 10- to 100-fold less RNA than that required with fluorescent probes using glass slides. This allows specific tissue samples or brain structures to be studied.

Figure 5.2 shows 10 µg of total RNA from a multiple sclerosis lesion hybridized to an array of >2400 cDNA targets on a glass microscope slide (Whitney et al., 1999). The spot spacing is approximately 450 µm, center to center. This slide was analyzed with ImageQuant software on a Amersham Biosciences STORM phosphoimager at 50 µm resolution.

**Two-Color Array Hybridization and Image Representation**
A disadvantage of the use of $^{33}$P-labeled probes on filters or glass slides is the inability to do a simultaneous two-color hybridization.

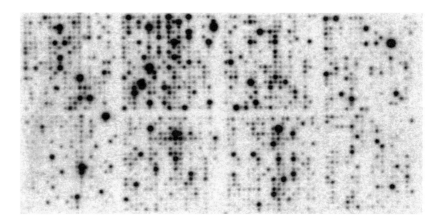

**Figure 5.2** Multiple sclerosis chronic lesion, 10 µg total RNA, glass array format.

The simultaneous two-sided hybridization approach is of value in some cases because it allows a direct comparison on the same set of targets. This is important when there is high variability between arrays. Simultaneous two-color hybridizations become less important with higher-quality control in array production, resulting in lower spot-to-spot variability. Different arrays become more easily compared with single probes that are either fluorescent or radiolabeled.

The steps involved in processing cDNA images to produce a two-color representation of array results are similar, if not identical, whether fluorescent or radioactive labels are used. Images from experiments using identically prepared arrays are digitally pseudo-colored and overlaid to produce a red-green composite image. This approach is similar for Cy3-, Cy5-, or $^{33}$P-labeled probes.

### Limiting Tissues and Experimental Approaches

Gene expression analysis in neural applications quite often focuses on small quantities of tissue from specific regions of the brain or isolated neural structures. The amount of tissue used for expression profiling can influence the cDNA array format used, the type of study performed, the method of probe labeling, and the interpretation of data.

Glass slides in combination with fluorescent probes (Cy3 and Cy5) have generally been used with cell lines (DeRisi et al., 1996; Khan et al., 1998) owing to the large amounts of total RNA needed (approximately 100–200 µg) when labeling with fluorescent-tagged nucleotides. A version of fluorescent probe labeling uses tyramide signal amplification (Perkin Elmer Life Sciences). This allows the use of RNA probes down to 2 µg of total RNA. However, this system requires an enzymatic amplification to generate a signal. While in most cases this enzymatic amplification is consistently linear, for some specific genes it is possible that such a step will introduce artifacts.

As mentioned earlier, [33]P-dCTP-labeled probes can be used at 1–10 µg total RNA. This is approximately the amount of total RNA found in 10–50 mg of brain tissue.

### Amplification of DNA or RNA Probes

As the amount of tissue, and thus the amount of RNA, used for expression profiling decreases from unlimited quantities to a single cell, different strategies have to be used to generate hybridization probes. There have been two general approaches used, antisense RNA (aRNA) amplification using T7 RNA polymerase (Crino et al., 1998; Kacharmina et al., 1999; Wang et al., 2000), and PCR. Both strategies produce amplified probes; however, PCR tends to skew the proportional representation of the final complex probe compared with the unamplified product. aRNA amplification is a more linear amplification and may be useful in certain applications. aRNA amplified probes can be used with either fluorescent or [33]P-labeled probes. Caution should be used with all cDNA amplification strategies since misrepresentation of the original RNA population could occur. aRNA amplification has been used in combination with laser capture microdissection (LCM) to study adjacent neuronal subtypes in rat brain (Luo et al., 1999).

Signal amplification is a potential alternative to nucleic acid amplification for limited probe preparation. It may be possible to use limiting quantities of cDNA or RNA probes in combination with quantitative methods of signal amplification, such as chemiluminescence or enzyme-linked signal amplification as discussed earlier (see also chapter 1).

### Cell Lines vs. Heterogeneous Tissues

Another major consideration in array-based experiments using neural tissue is the heterogeneity of the tissue studied. In many cases, a cell line or homogeneous tissue is used and thus the reproducibility and interpretation of the experiment is straightforward. Some of the emerging broad-based quantitative statistical approaches to array-based gene expression may be used. However, in other cases, the main application of cDNA arrays in conjunction with heterogeneous tissue may be as a simple large-scale primary screen for changes in RNA expression. This places a stronger emphasis on downstream validation assays such as *in situ* hybridization, quantitative PCR, immunohistochemistry, RNA dot blots, RNase protection, and traditional Northern blot analysis compared with array-based experiments using cell lines or homogeneous tissues. Downstream experimental validation also may provide cell type specificity and anatomical context relevant to neuroscience applications.

Similarly, results from whole-array-based statistical quantitative methods (Eisen et al., 1998; Bassett et al., 1999) are less clear using heterogeneous tissues, since apparent quantitative RNA changes may be due to differences in cell types or cell number and not to de novo initiation of gene transcription.

The ability to acquire samples and make appropriate complex probes from limited amounts of tissue addresses some issues of cellular complexity. Techniques such as laser capture microdissection (Bonner et al., 1997) or aRNA amplification (Crino et al., 1998; Kacharmina et al., 1999) have been useful in reducing the complexity of heterogeneous tissues to prepare specific probes for cDNA arrays.

An additional strategy when working with heterogeneous tissues is to perform a series of reduction screenings in a fashion similar to traditional cDNA library screening. That is, (1) use an initial large array-based screen to identify many candidate changes, (2) go back to the original library and isolate positive clones, (3) make a large number of subarrays and confirm the original RNA changes.

## Conclusion

Large-scale gene expression techniques are rapidly having an impact in many areas of biomedical research. Neuroscience applications of cDNA arrays and array-based technologies require special considerations. Primarily these include the use of complex heterogeneous tissues and limited amounts of tissues, and the related issues of interpreting complex data. Since genomic-scale assays are being applied with greater frequency and success to problems using neural tissue, long-standing questions may be addressed concerning neurodegeneration, psychiatric and developmental disorders, and other molecular questions in the brain.

## Acknowledgments

The authors would like to thank Drs. Mark Vawter, Chris Cheadle, William H. Wood III, and Dave Donovan for helpful suggestions.

**Protocol:** Radioactive labeling

The following is a brief RNA-to-cDNA radioactive labeling protocol for both membrane and glass arrays.

1. Mix 1 μg of oligo-dT oligonucleotide (Invitrogen Poly T) and 5–10 μg of total RNA in diethyl pyrocarbonate (DEPC)-$H_2O$ in a 0.5-ml microfuge tube.

2. Add $H_2O$ to 15 µl, heat to 70 °C for 10 minutes, place on ice 2 minutes.
3. To this reaction add:
   8 µl 5× first-strand buffer (LTI #18084-014)
   4 µl 0.1 M dithiothreitol (DTT) (LTI #18084-014)
   4 µl 3 dNTPs mixture (0.5 mM each minus dCTP [Pharmacia #27-20X0])
   1 µl RNAseOUT (LTI #18084-014)
   5 µl $^{33}$P-$\alpha$-dCTP (ICN #58430)
   $H_2O$ up to 38 µl total volume.
4. To this mixture, add 2 µl SSII reverse transcriptase (LTI #18084-014); incubate at 42 °C for 35 minutes.
5. Add an additional 2 µl SSII RT and incubate at 42 °C for 35 minutes.
6. Add 5 µl 0.5 M EDTA and 10 µl 0.1 N NaOH; incubate at 65 °C for 30 minutes.
7. Add 25 µl 1 M Tris HCl, pH 8.0.
8. Prepare a Biospin P-30 spin column (Bio-Rad #732-6223) as per manufacturer's instructions.
9. Load the entire sample on column and spin.
10. Recover approximately a 75 µl sample.
11. Count 1 µl in a scintillation counter.

**Membrane hybridization**

1. Load microfilters into 50-ml conical tubes, "dot side" inward.
2. Prewash microfilters in 2× SSC for 5 minutes.
3. Add 4 ml Microhyb (Invitrogen #HYB250.GF) prewarmed to 50 °C.
4. Heat denature the following three blocking agents at 95 °C for 5 minutes before adding:
   100 µl human $C_0t$-1 DNA (LTI #15279-001), 100 µl poly A at 8 mg/ml (Sigma #P-9403), 40 µl sheared salmon sperm DNA at 10 mg/ml.
5. Prehybridize, rotating at 50 °C, at least 4 hours.
6. Heat denature the probe (approximately 75 µl) at 95 °C for 5 minutes.
7. Add the probe (~75 µl) (probe count should be *at least* $1 \times 10^6$ count/ml hybridization solution).
8. Hybridize at 50 °C, rotating overnight (16–18 hours).

**Washing conditions**

1. Do a quick wash in the hybridization tube with approximately 50 ml wash solution 1 (2× SSC and 0.1% SDS).
2. Continue washes at room temperature with 50 ml wash solution 1 with shaking. (Wash two times at room temperature in wash solution 1 for 10 minutes each. Survey the filters with a radioactive survey meter, and if necessary, continue washing.)

3. Wash two times at room temperature in wash solution 2 ($1\times$ SSC and 0.1% SDS) for 15 minutes each. The exact extent of washing must be determined empirically.

## Exposure

1. Place wet membranes, "dot side up" on a clean dry glass plate.
2. Place a strip of wet filter paper on the bottom of the glass plate for humidity control.
3. Cover the plate with plastic wrap.
4. Pull plastic wrap *very tightly* and tape to the back of the plate. Smooth out *all* microbubbles. Small variations on a microscale look very large.
5. Place plate in bleached phosphoimager cassette.
6. Expose the membranes overnight, then scan on an Amersham Biosciences STORM phosphoimager set to 50-μm resolution.
7. Empirically determine the need for a longer exposure (anywhere from 3 to 10 days).

## Stripping of membranes

1. Wash two times at 65 °C in 0.4 N NaOH/0.1% SDS for 30 minutes each in ~200–300-ml solution with vigorous shaking.
2. Wash two times at room temperature in 0.2 M Tris HCl (pH 8.0)/$1\times$ SSC/0.1% SDS for 10 minutes each.
3. Air dry and expose to a phosphor screen overnight to determine stripping efficiency. Membranes can be reused three to five times.

## Note

1. For a protocol for labeling cDNA with [33]P-dCTP for use on glass slides, see http://www.nhgri.nih.gov/DIR/LCG/15K/HTML/protocol.html

## References

Barrett T, Cheadle C, Wood WH, Teichberg D, Donovan DM, Freed WJ, Becker KG, and Vawter MP (2001). Assembly and use of a broadly applicable neural cDNA microarray. *Restorative Neurology and Neuroscience* 18: 127–35.
Bassett DE Jr, Eisen MB, and Boguski MS (1999). Gene expression informatics—it's all in your mine. *Nat Genet* 21(Suppl. 1): 51–5.
Bertucci F, Bernard K, Loriod B, Chang YC, Granjeaud S, Birnbaum D, Nguyen C, Peck K, and Jordan BR (1999). Sensitivity issues in DNA array-based expression measure-

ments and performance of nylon microarrays for small samples. *Human Mol Genet* 8(9): 1715–22.

Bonner RF, Emmert-Buck M, Cole K, Pohida T, Chuaqui R, Goldstein S, and Liotta LA (1997). Laser capture microdissection: Molecular analysis of tissue. *Science* 278(5342): 1481, 1483.

Chen JJ, Wu R, Yang PC, Huang JY, Sher YP, Han MH, Kao WC, Lee PJ, Chiu TF, Chang F, Chu YW, Wu CW, and Peck K (1998). Profiling expression patterns and isolating differentially expressed genes by cDNA microarray system with colorimetry detection. *Genomics* 51: 313–24.

Crino P, Khodakhah K, Becker K, Ginsberg S, Hemby S, and Eberwine J (1998). Presence and phosphorylation of transcription factors in developing dendrites. *Proc Natl Acad Sci USA* 95(5): 2313–18.

DeRisi J, Penland L, Brown PO, Bittner ML, Meltzer PS, Ray M, Chen Y, Su YA, and Trent JM (1996). Use of a cDNA microarray to analyse gene expression patterns in human cancer. *Nat Genet* 14: 457–60.

Duggan DJ, Bittner M, Chen Y, Meltzer P, and Trent JM (1999). Expression profiling using cDNA microarrays. *Nat Genet* 21(Suppl. 1): 10–14.

Dunham I, Shimizu N, Roe BA, Chissoe S, Hunt AR, Collins JE, Bruskiewich R, Beare DM, Clamp M, Smink LJ, Ainscough R, Almeida JP, Babbage A, Bagguley C, Bailey J, Barlow K, Bates KN, Beasley O, Bird CP, Blakey S, Bridgeman AM, Buck D, Burgess J, Burrill WD, O'Brien KP, et al. (1999). The DNA sequence of human chromosome 22. *Nature* 402(6761): 489–95.

Eisen MB, Spellman PT, Brown PO, and Botstein D (1998). Cluster analysis and display of genome-wide expression patterns. *Proc Natl Acad Sci USA* 95(25): 14863–8.

Ewing B and Green P (2000). Analysis of expressed sequence tags indicates 35,000 human genes. *Nat Genet* 25(2): 232–4.

Hattori M, Fujiyama A, Taylor TD, Watanabe H, Yada T, Park HS, Toyoda A, Ishii K, Totoki Y, Choi DK, Soeda E, Ohki M, Takagi T, Sakaki Y, Taudien S, Blechschmidt K, Polley A, Menzel U, Delabar J, Kumpf K, Lehmann R, Patterson D, Reichwald K, Rump A, Schillhabel M, and Schudy A (2000). The DNA sequence of human chromosome 21. The chromosome 21 mapping and sequencing consortium. *Nature* 405(6784): 311–19.

Kacharmina JE, Crino PB, and Eberwine J (1999). Preparation of cDNA from single cells and subcellular regions. *Methods Enzymol* 303: 3–18.

Khan J, Simon R, Bittner M, Chen Y, Leighton SB, Pohida T, Smith PD, Jiang Y, Gooden GC, Trent JM, and Meltzer PS (1998). Gene expression profiling of alveolar rhabdomyosarcoma with cDNA microarrays. *Cancer Res* 58(22): 5009–13.

Lipshutz RJ, Fodor SP, Gingeras TR, and Lockhart DJ (1999). High-density synthetic oligonucleotide arrays. *Nat Genet* 21(Suppl. 1): 20–4.

Luo L, Salunga RC, Guo H, Bittner A, Joy KC, Galindo JE, Xiao H, Rogers KE, Wan JS, Jackson MR, and Erlander MG (1999). Gene expression profiles of laser-captured adjacent neuronal subtypes. *Nat Med* 5(1): 117–22.

Pietu G, Alibert O, Guichard V, Lamy B, Bois F, Leroy E, Mariage-Sampson R, Houlgatte R, Soularue P, and Auffray C (1996). Novel gene transcripts preferentially expressed in human muscles revealed by quantitative hybridization of a high density cDNA array. *Genome Res* 6(6): 492–503.

Sargent TD and Dawid IB (1983). Differential gene expression in the gastrula of *Xenopus laevis*. *Science* 222(4620): 135–9.

Schena M, Shalon D, Davis RW, and Brown PO (1995). Quantitative monitoring of gene expression patterns with a complementary DNA microarray. *Science* 270(5235): 467–70.

Tanaka TS, Jaradet SA, Lim MK, Kargul GJ, Wang X, Grahovac MJ, Pantano S, Sano Y, Piao Y, Nagaraja R, Doi H, Wood WH, Becker KG, and Ko MSH (2000). Genome-wide expression profiling of mid-gestation placenta and embryo using a 15K mouse developmental cDNA microarray. *Proc Natl Acad Sci USA* 97(16): 9127–32.

Vawter MP, Barrett T, Cheadle C, Sokolov BP, Wood WH III, Donovan DM, Webster M, Freed WJ, and Becker KG (2001). Application of cDNA microarrays to examine gene expression differences in schizophrenia. *Brain Research Bulletin* 55(5): 641–50.

Wang E, Miller LD, Ohnmacht GA, Liu ET, and Marincola FM (2000). High-fidelity mRNA amplification for gene profiling. *Nat Biotechnol* 18: 457–9.

Whitney LW and Becker KG (2001). Radioactive [33]P probes in hybridization to glass cDNA microarrays using neural tissues. *J Neurosci Methods* 106(1): 9–13.

Whitney LW, Becker KG, Tresser NJ, Caballero-Ramos CI, Munson PJ, Prabhu VV, Trent JM, McFarland HF, and Biddison WE (1999). Analysis of gene expression in mutiple sclerosis lesions using cDNA microarrays. *Ann Neurol* 46(3): 425–8.

Zhao N, Hashida H, Takahashi N, Misumi Y, and Sakaki Y (1995). High-density cDNA filter analysis: A novel approach for large-scale, quantitative analysis of gene expression. *Gene* 156(2): 207–13.

# 6   Custom-Built cDNA Arrays for the Study of Neuronal Differentiation and Disease: The Smart Chip

*Lillian W. Chiang, Dave Ficenec, and Jill M. Grenier*

Comparative hybridization of RNA samples on high-density cDNA microarrays has been successfully used to characterize genome-scale mRNA expression in a variety of basic cellular processes. Global RNA regulation during cellular processes such as cell-cycle regulation (Cho et al., 1998; Spellman et al., 1998), fibroblast growth control (Iyer et al., 1999), metabolic responses to growth medium (DeRisi et al., 1997), and germ cell development (Chu et al., 1998) have been temporally monitored using cDNA arrays. The program of gene expression delineated in these studies demonstrates a correlation between shared functional pathways and temporally coupled expression. Clustering of temporal expression profiles for known genes provided a dynamic overall picture of the cell biology involved (reviewed by Brown and Botstein, 1999).

Steps to deriving such relevant insights from expression profiling include experimental design, clone selection, method optimization, data analysis, and data interpretation. Whether one chooses glass, nylon, oligonucleotide-based, or other array technologies, a significant amount of resources are utilized, including precious tissue and/or cell samples in addition to equipment and reagents. Because the data obtained are information intensive, careful consideration of data filtering mechanisms is warranted. This chapter discusses experimental design issues with regard to clone selection for a brain-biased and a dorsal root ganglia (DRG)-biased array, as well as method optimization, with nylon technology as an example. The advantages of nylon technology include accessibility and sensitivity, but mostly we chose it to facilitate the arraying of custom clone sets.

In yeast, the complete genome has been arrayed for expression-profiling experiments (Lashkari et al., 1997; Wodicka et al., 1997). In higher eukaryotes, the absence of a completed genome has necessitated arraying as many sequences as possible from known genes, from expressed sequence tags, or from uncharacterized cDNA clones from a library (reviewed by Bowtell, 1999; Duggan et al., 1999; Marshall and Hodgson, 1998; Ramsay, 1998). In most cases, practically achievable array element densities limit the number of genes that may be profiled relative to the amount of sample material (i.e., RNA) required.

Furthermore, as long as the relevant genes are represented, having fewer array elements facilitates certain data and statistical analyses, and minimizes data storage requirements. Therefore, clone selection methods have been used to enrich for differentially expressed or paradigm-relevant genes; these methods include differential display (Luo et al., 1999), library subtraction (Geschwind et al., 2001; see also chapter 10 by Geschwind and Nelson), and selection of informatics (Loftus et al., 1999).

By querying the public EST database (dbEST), Loftus and colleagues first used an informatics approach to identify an EST library that was particularly rich for melanocyte markers. They then arrayed clones from the identified library and demonstrated by expression profiling that many more of the genes represented were differentially expressed between melanoma and kidney epithelial cell lines than with clones arrayed from an unselected library.

In the method described in this chapter, we constructed and sequenced custom cDNA libraries first and then used an informatics approach to select nonredundant ESTs for preparing array elements. The resulting array, designated the Smart Chip, was designed for the study of neuronal disease and differentiation. However, the approach can be generalized to any particular neurobiological system of interest.

As outlined in this chapter, the construction and validation of custom arrays involves the following steps: (1) application of informatics approaches to select clones of interest; (2) use of a robotic sampler to consolidate and sequence selected clones; (3) optimization of hybridization conditions for sensitivity, reproducibility, and dynamic range; (4) validation of expression profiling results by reverse-transcriptase polymerase chain reaction (RT-PCR); and (5) characterization of nervous system-specific gene expression.

## Clone Set Design

Our initial goal was to assemble an array specifically enriched for genes involved in neurodegeneration in the central nervous system (Chiang et al., 2001). At the time, a limited number of rat sequences were available, so we sequenced our own cDNA libraries and used an informatics approach to remove redundancy within the libraries. Subsequently, we wished to increase the diversity of novel genes represented relevant to diseases of the peripheral nervous system (PNS). Since the rat sequences in the public databases at this later time were significantly more numerous than when we started, we modified our informatics approach to utilize this new information to further reduce the redundancy and also to increase the novelty of the selected clones.

### Initial Enrichment for Genes Involved in Neurodegeneration

Two cDNA libraries were generated. One was from the rat frontal cortex, to enrich for genes expressed in the central nervous system, and the other was from differentiated PC12 cells deprived of nerve growth factor (NGF), to enrich for genes upregulated during neuronal differentiation and to provide a model of neuronal programmed cell death (Rukenstein et al., 1991). Expressed sequence tags were determined for the 5′-end of cDNA clones picked from both libraries. To minimize the redundancy of the clones arrayed, 7399 out of 13,984 ESTs from these two libraries were determined to be representative of unique genes by sequence comparison analysis (figure 6.1A). Sequence comparisons were done using the Basic Local Alignment Search Tool (BLAST) (Altschul et al., 1990). Con-

A.

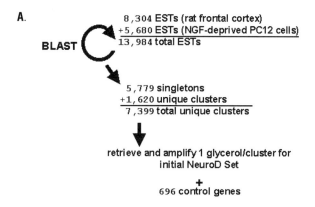

8,304 ESTs (rat frontal cortex)
+5,680 ESTs (NGF-deprived PC12 cells)
13,984 total ESTs

BLAST

5,779 singletons
+1,620 unique clusters
7,399 total unique clusters

retrieve and amplify 1 glycerol/cluster for
initial NeuroD Set
+
696 control genes

B.

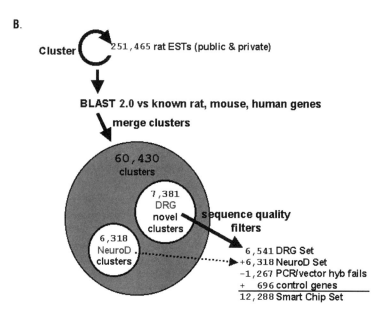

Cluster 251,465 rat ESTs (public & private)

BLAST 2.0 vs known rat, mouse, human genes
merge clusters

60,430 clusters

7,381
DRG
novel
clusters

sequence quality
filters

6,318
NeuroD
clusters

6,541 DRG Set
+6,318 NeuroD Set
-1,267 PCR/vector hyb fails
+    696 control genes
12,288 Smart Chip Set

**Figure 6.1**   Strategies for designing Smart Chip clone sets. (*A*) Enrichment for genes involved in neurodegeneration (NeuroD) was achieved by sequencing two relevant cDNA libraries: one from rat frontal cortex, the other from NGF-deprived differentiated PC12 cells. BLAST was used to cluster the sequences within these two libraries. One representative clone was chosen from each unique cluster for arraying along with 696 control genes. (*B*) Enrichment for novel genes expressed in DRG was achieved by clustering all available rat ESTs (public and private). Consensus contigs of each cluster were compared with known rat, mouse, and human genes. The remaining novel clusters included 7381 that contained ESTs from an axotomized DRG library, and 6318 that contained ESTs from the original NeuroD set. After a sequence quality filter was applied, and PCR and vector hybridization quality control were performed, a total of 12,288 comprised the clones arrayed on the Smart Chip.

tiguous matches (contigs) defined a sequence cluster. Large clusters were checked by hand to eliminate apparent chimeras.

From 13,984 sequences, the analysis identified 5779 singletons (only one EST in the cluster) and 1620 larger clusters. All of the singletons and one representative clone from each large cluster were chosen for arraying. In addition to the ESTs, 696 known genes were also selected, such as those with known function in the CNS, housekeeping genes, and negative hybridization controls such as vector, poly A, or $C_0t$-1 sequences (table 6.1).

### Subsequent Enrichment for Novel Genes Expressed in DRG

A total of 46,288 ESTs were determined from a rat cDNA library constructed from RNA isolated and pooled from rat DRG at 1, 3, 7, 14, and 21 days after axotomy. For the second version of the clone set, we used a comprehensive EST clustering system incorporating CAT 3.2 (Cluster Analysis Tools; www.DoubleTwist.com) as the engine to cluster the 46,288 DRG ESTs with all known ESTs (public and private, totaling 251,465) (figure 6.1B).

To further reduce redundancy, the contigs (obtained from assembly of the EST clusters) were clustered by sequence similarity to known mRNA sequences from rat, mouse, and human. A match required an overlap of 150 bases and at least 95% identity for rat and mouse and 90% identity for human. WU-BLAST 2.0 (Altschul et al., 1990), which allows for gapped alignments, was used.

The result was 60,430 clusters, of which 6318 contained ESTs from the initial neurodegeneration set. The remaining 54,112 contained 7381 clusters unique to the axotomized DRG library. In other words, the ESTs comprising these 7381 contigs were only found in our DRG library. Since 6532 clusters were singletons, 400 were selected at random and analyzed by hand to assess the quality. Ten percent appeared to be of poor quality (short sequence or high fraction of ambiguous calls); 20% appeared to represent false singletons since significant hits to rat gene sequences were found by BLAST; the remaining 70% were assumed to be true rat

**Table 6.1** Smart Chip control array elements

| CONTROL ARRAY ELEMENT(S) | DESCRIPTION |
|---|---|
| poly(dA)$_{>200}$ | Since most of the ESTs were poly A$^+$, important negative control tests stringency of hybridization. |
| 5'-end, middle, and 3'-end actin, glial fibrillary acidic protein (GFAP), and reduced glyceraldehyde-phosphate dehydrogenase (GAPDH) fragments | Relative signals indicate quality of labeled probe as reflected by length. |
| Rat, human, mouse genomic and C$_0t$ DNA | Robust signals to these negative controls indicate nonspecific hybridization to low-entropy sequences found in 10–15% of all cDNAs. |
| *E. coli*, plasmid, and lambda genomic DNA | Negative controls test for vector contamination in the labeled probe. |
| Known apoptosis genes | e.g., XIAP, Bcl-2, caspases. |
| CNS markers | e.g., synaptotagmin, α CaMKII. |
| PNS markers | e.g., galanin, CGRP, preprodynorphin. |
| Other genes | e.g., paradigm-specific genes, *c-fos*, HSPs, S100β, neuronal enolase, neurofilament, vimentin. |
| Duplicate control sets | A subset of controls exactly duplicated on both filters of the complete Smart Chip array set facilitates intrafilter set normalization. |
| tRNAs and rRNAs | Especially important for total RNA samples, these negative controls indicate extent of labeling of non-poly A$^+$ RNAs. |
| Replicate actin array elements | Multiple identical actin array elements spaced throughout the array, especially in the corners, aid in orienting the array grid for densitometry, and also indicate overall consistency of array element deposition and hybridization. |

singletons. Therefore we added automated steps to eliminate short or poor-quality sequences in the 7381 cluster contig sequences. Requirements were that they be at least 250 bases in length and contain less than 5% ambiguous calls. From the resulting set of 6541 clusters, a representative clone was chosen from each cluster in such a manner as to minimize the number of plates retrieved for consolidation.

### Clone Set Consolidation and Quality Control of Array Element

A major challenge in constructing custom clone sets is ensuring high-fidelity tracking of the sequences to the clones and to the array elements. Using a Genesis RSP 150 robotic sample processor (Tecan AG, Switzerland) and a Qbot multitasking robot (Genetix, United Kingdom), bacterial cultures of individual EST clones from the libraries were consolidated from 60,080 clones spanning more than 600 microtiter plates to 12,859 clones spanning 134 microtiter plates.

To prepare templates to be array elements, oligonucleotide primers flanking the cloning site of the library vector were used to PCR amplify the cDNA insert present in each bacterial culture (see protocol 1 at the end of the chapter). The conditions were optimized, resulting in 85–90% successful amplification as assessed by detection of a single band by ethidium bromide staining after agarose gel electrophoresis.

In addition, we routinely performed a "vector hybridization" utilizing a radiolabeled DNA probe that is homologous to the vector sequences common to all of the array elements (figure 6.2). Complete failure of the PCR was easily detected by this method. We eliminated those bacterial clones that consistently failed to PCR amplify by reconsolidating with the robotic sample processor. The remaining 12,288 PCR templates were arrayed onto nylon filters, resulting in a two-filter Smart Chip set containing 6144 elements each (protocol 1).

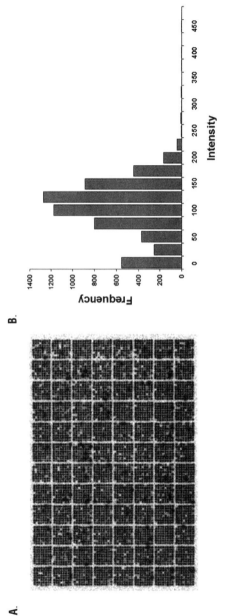

**Figure 6.2** Smart Chip characterization by vector hybridization. (*A*) Approximately 200 nucleotides flanking the multiple cloning site of the library vector common to all array templates were amplified by PCR. After agarose gel purification, the PCR product was radiolabeled using a Prime-It room temperature random primer labeling kit (Stratagene, La Jolla, Calif.). Arrays were hybridized with the radiolabeled PCR probe at 65 °C, as described in protocol 2, for 3.5 hours. The image shown was taken after a 16-hour exposure to a phosphoimage screen. (*B*) Hybridization signals by the PCR probe to the array elements shown in (*A*) were quantified by densitometry and grouped into bins by intensity. For all values, 85% fell in a tight 50–300 intensity range. Consistent with the observed failure rate of array element PCR, <10% fell in the "0" intensity bin.

Since we were interested in understanding the cell biology of the paradigms profiled as well as identifying new genes, the tracking fidelity of array elements was critical for correctly annotating Smart Chip ESTs with significant homology to known genes. Therefore, a statistically significant subset of the ESTs consolidated and arrayed was chosen randomly for sequence validation. All 202 successfully sequenced clones matched their seed sequence, implying 100% fidelity.

**Hybridization**

The three components of method optimization for any nucleic acid hybridization are reproducibility, sensitivity, and specificity. Intra-array reproducibility can be affected by inconsistency of array element deposition and densitometry. Sensitivity can be affected by the efficiency of the RNA probe labeling and signal-to-background noise. Specificity can be affected by the stringency of hybridization conditions and washes.

Using optimal labeling, hybridization, and wash conditions worked out for nylon arrays (see protocol 2 at the end of the chapter), radiolabeled cDNA hybridized to triplicate arrays was detected and quantified by digitizing the phosphoimager-captured signal intensity for each gene. Reproducibility as reflected by the coefficient of variation was quite good, averaging less than 0.2 for spots whose intensities were above threshold (figure 6.3). The dynamic range of detection spanned three orders of magnitude. We exposed the filters so that the gene expression intensity for the most abundant messages barely saturated the phosphoimager screens. In this manner, with the described protocols, the signal-to-noise ratio was such that we were able to detect the less abundant genes that would otherwise have been below the detection threshold. From control experiments in which *in vitro* transcribed RNAs were spiked into samples, this detection threshold amounted to a copy number of less than 1 in 100,000 (data not shown).

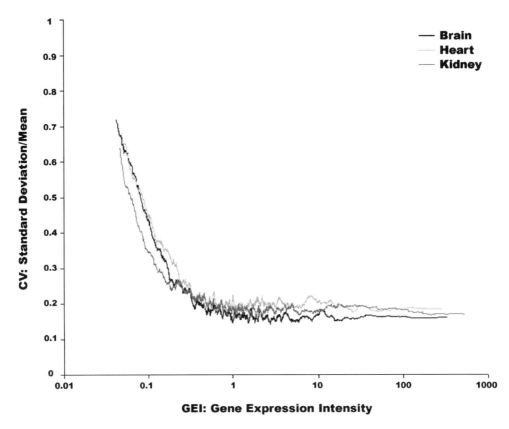

**Figure 6.3**  Reproducibility between array hybridizations. After normalization, the coefficient of variation (standard deviation/average gene expression intensity) for each array element (12,288 total) was plotted against the mean intensity for the gene (GEI). The average was graphed for three different mRNA probes made from rat brain, heart, and kidney. The average CV above an intensity of 1 was 0.2 or below for all probes.

### RT-PCR Validation

Although the reproducibility in expression profiling experiments was high, the apparent mRNA regulation of known and novel genes was validated by another method in order to test specificity. Semiquantitative RT-PCR was chosen for several reasons, including sensitivity, throughput, and specificity. Since expression profiling is essentially a Southern blotting technique, possible artifacts that may arise include detection of signals generated as a result of stable hybrids forming between closely related nucleic acids such as splice variants, isoforms, or even closely related protein family members.

For each gene, semiquantitative RT-PCR results were interpreted as an indication of its expression as upregulated, downregulated, or unchanged. This was done by comparing the dilution at which the RT-PCR product was no longer visible on ethidium bromide-stained gels between control and treated samples. For example, in figure 6.4, neuronal enolase was not regulated by "treatment," whereas *c-jun* and caspase 3 were upregulated, and *c-fos* was downregulated. For 51 genes assayed by this method, the regulation observed by expression profiling for 41 genes was validated, implying approximately 20% false positives. Given the high reproducibility observed between triplicate hybridizations (average CV = 0.2), the false positives detected by RT-PCR are likely due to cross-hybridization by mRNAs with homologous or related genes.

A high failure rate among the RT-PCR primers designed was observed; 65 out of 161 primers used resulted in undetectable product or a smear. The design of 57 out of the 65 failed primers was based on the original EST as opposed to a base-perfect finished sequence of selected array elements, indicating that PCR failure was likely due to the poor sequence quality of ESTs. Out of 31 array elements for which a base-perfect sequence was obtained, the average insert size was 1850 bp and 7 contained full-length open reading frames. Only one finished sequence did not match its seed EST.

## Characterization of Nervous System-Specific Gene Expression

To characterize the tissue distribution of genes on the Smart Chip and to identify brain- and/or DRG-specific genes, we hybridized radiolabeled cDNA prepared from fourteen different normal rat tissues. These included rat brain, heart, kidney, liver, lung, pancreas, skeletal muscle, smooth muscle, spleen, testes, DRG, sciatic nerve, spinal cord, and skin. As expected, radiolabeled brain

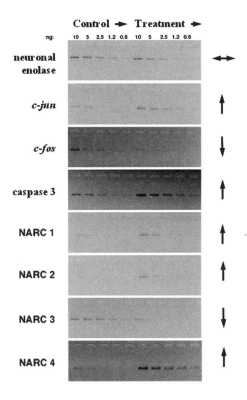

**Figure 6.4** RT-PCR validation of expression profiling results. Oligonucleotide primer sequences specific for each EST were designed with a melting temperature of 55–60 °C as predicted by PrimerSelect software (DNASTAR, Inc., Madison, Wis.). A Stratagene Opti-Prime kit was used to optimize RT-PCR for each primer pair. Reactions on twofold serially diluted control and treated cDNA were set up robotically (Genesis RSP 150) to ensure high-fidelity assembly and to automatically incorporate the distinct optimal buffer for each primer pair. Every robot run included primers specific for housekeeping genes, such as neuronal enolase to control for template dilutions. The number of cycles was adjusted to obtain a linear range of amplification. Regulation of *c-jun*, *c-fos*, and caspase 3 was determined by comparing the dilution at which RT-PCR product was no longer visible between control and withdrawn samples.

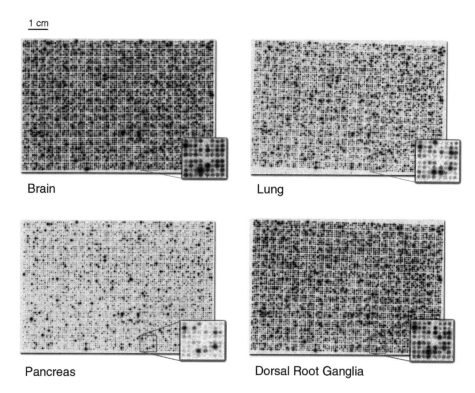

1 cm

Brain

Lung

Pancreas

Dorsal Root Ganglia

**Figure 6.5** Organ hybridization filter images. Shown are the images of filters containing 6144 Smart Chip array elements hybridized to rat brain, lung, pancreas, and DRG cDNA, with brain tissue exhibiting a detectable signal for most of the elements.

cDNA hybridized more intensely to most of the array elements than some of the other non-neuronal tissues tested (figure 6.5). In fact, consistent with our selection criteria, 114 and 103 genes appeared to be brain and DRG specific, respectively, compared with the non-neuronal tissues tested (table 6.2). Most (11,254 out of 12,000) but not all of the ESTs were detected in at least one of the tissues profiled (table 6.2). Since we eliminated most of the poorly amplified array clones through a reconsolidation step, those array elements producing no signal may have represented cDNA clones whose inserts were too small to form stable hybrids, or ESTs that

**Table 6.2** Tissue distribution of Smart Chip array elements

| CATEGORY/TISSUE | NO. OF EST ARRAY ELEMENTS |
| --- | --- |
| Total EST array elements | 12,000 |
| Detected in any tissue[a] | 11,254 |
| Detected in the nervous system (brain, DRG, spinal cord, sciatic nerve, or skin) | 10,589 |
| Detected in brain | 9893 |
| Detected in DRG | 9885 |
| Detected in brain and DRG | 9475 |
| Detected in all tissues | 8092 |
| Brain-specific expression[b] | 114 |
| Heart-specific expression | 24 |
| Testes-specific expression | 81 |
| Kidney-specific expression | 5 |
| DRG-specific expression | 103 |

[a]Fourteen tissues were tested: rat brain, heart, kidney, liver, lung, pancreas, skeletal muscle, smooth muscle, spleen, testes, DRG, sciatic nerve, spinal cord, and skin. The number detected was tabulated as the number of array elements producing a GEI greater than 1.
[b]Brain-, heart-, testes- and kidney-specific genes were determined by comparing expression in ten tissues: brain, heart, kidney, liver, lung, pancreas, skeletal muscle, smooth muscle, spleen, and testes. DRG-specific genes were determined by comparison with the same tissues except brain.

are expressed at levels below the detection threshold in all the tissues tested.

## Summary

Having demonstrated the novelty and the nervous system bias of genes represented on the Smart Chip, multiple studies to understand transcriptional regulation during neuronal differentiation, programmed cell death, and disease have been initiated. In many of the paradigms investigated, ischemia, for example, up to 1700 genes on the Smart Chip were significantly regulated more than threefold.

As discussed in other chapters, software that supports the archiving, annotation, and analysis of the data is critical for interpretation of such information-intensive experiments. In addition, profiling of multiple experimental models, time points, and/or dose responses allows one to subcategorize the regulated genes by experimental overlap, temporal regulation, and/or dose dependence in expression patterns.

Given the resources and effort required, careful consideration of the genes profiled using custom arrays contributes to the thoroughness of the gene expression screen. Even as genome-scale arrays become available for higher eukaryotes, smaller paradigm-specific arrays may be desirable for throughput analyses in specific model organisms.

## Acknowledgments

We would like to thank Keith Robison for BLAST analysis; Fenyu Jin for Smart Chip consolidation; and Millennium core groups— cDNA libraries, sequencing, process technology, informatics and TRACE—for library construction, EST sequencing, data acquisition, software, and array production.

**Protocol 1:** Preparation and deposition of array elements

1. Using oligonucleotide primers flanking the cloning site of the cDNA inserts, perform PCR directly on bacterial cultures containing each EST as recommended by Ab Peptides, Inc. (St. Louis, Mo.).

**Reagents**
4 µl       bacterial culture
10.5 µl    10 × PC2 buffer (from Ab Peptides without bovine serum albumin, BSA)
1.05 µl    40 µM forward primer

    1.05 μl   40 μM reverse primer
    1.05 μl   20 mM dNTPs (each at 5 mM)
    0.5 μl   KlenTaq1 DNA polymerase (Ab Peptides, Inc.)
    Add $H_2O$ to 100 μl.

2. Ethanol precipitate and concentrate amplified array templates in 3× SSC to 1–10 mg/ml.

3. Array 20 nl onto nylon filters (Biodyne B, Gibco BRL Life Technologies, Gaithersburg, Md.) at a density of ~64/cm$^2$ using a 96-well format pin robot (CRS Robotics, Burlington, Ontario, Canada). Allow filters to dry completely.

4. Denature filters in 0.4 M NaOH.

5. Neutralize filters in 0.1 M Tris HCl, pH 7.5.

6. Rinse filters in 2× SSC.

7. Dry filters completely for use in hybridizations.

**Solutions**

1× SSC:
150 mM sodium chloride
15 mM sodium citrate, pH 7.0

1× PC2:
50 mM Tris HCl, pH 9.1
16 mM ammonium sulfate
3.5 mM $MgCl_2$

**Protocol 2:**  Probe preparation, array hybridization, and image capture

1. First-strand cDNA synthesis. Incubate the following at 50 °C for 30 minutes:

**Reagents**
RNA sample (1 μg poly A$^+$ or 10 μg total)
1 μg oligo(dT)$_{30}$
0.5 mM each dATP, dGTP, dTTP
100 μCi $^{33}$P-dCTP (2000–4000 Ci/mmol; NEN Life Science Products, Boston, Mass.)
40 U RNase inhibitor (Boehringer Mannheim, Germany)
200 U SSCII (Gibco BRL Life Technologies)
Add $H_2O$ to 20 μl.

2. Remove unincorporated deoxynucleotides using Chroma Spin +TE-30 column (Clontech, Palo Alto, Calif.).

3. Place two filters, separated by nylon mesh, into one 150-mm hybridization bottle (Robbins Scientific, Sunnyvale, Calif.). Add 10 ml preannealing solution carefully, avoiding the creation of bubbles. Preanneal for 1 hour at 65 °C in a rotating incubator (Robbins Scientific).
4. While arrays are preannealing, dilute radiolabeled first-strand cDNA probe. For two filters per hybridization bottle:
   $2 \times 10^7$ cpm probe
   10 µg poly(dA)$_{>200}$ (Amersham Pharmacia Biotech, Piscataway, N.J.)
   10 µg rat $C_0t$ 10 DNA (prepared as described by Britten et al., 1974)
   Add $H_2O$ to 100 µl
   Anneal at 65 °C for 4 hours.
5. Add probe mixture to preannealed arrays and hybridize overnight at 65 °C.
6. Wash twice with 2× SSC, 1% SDS for 15 minutes at 65 °C.
7. Wash twice with 0.2× SSC, 0.5% SDS for 30 minutes at 65 °C.
8. Wash twice with 2× SSC for 15 minutes at 22 °C. Dry array filters to completion.
9. Expose filters to phosphoimage screens (Fuji Medical Systems, Stamford, Conn.) for approximately 60 hours. Capture and digitize images with a Fuji BAS 2500 phosphoimager (Fuji Medical Systems). Quantitate images by densitometry using Array Vision software (Imaging Research Inc., Canada).

**Solutions**

PREANNEALING SOLUTION:
100 mg/ml sheared salmon sperm DNA
7% SDS
0.25 M sodium phosphate pH 7.2
1 mM EDTA
10% formamide

# References

Altschul SF, Gish W, Miller W, Myers EW, and Lipman DJ (1990). Basic local alignment search tool. *J Mol Biol* 215: 403–10.

Bowtell DDL (1999). Options available—from start to finish—for obtaining expression data by microarray. *Nat Genet* 21: 25–32.

Britten RJ, Graham DE, and Neufeld BR (1974). Analysis of repeating DNA sequences by reassociation. *Methods Enzymol* 29: 363–418.

Brown PO and Botstein D (1999). Exploring the new world of the genome with DNA microarrays. *Nat Genet* 21: 33–7.

Chiang LW, Grenier JM, Ettwiller L, Jenkins LP, Ficenec D, Martin J, Jin F, DiStefano PS, and Wood A (2001). An orchestrated gene expression component of neuronal programmed cell death revealed by cDNA array analysis. *Proc Natl Acad Sci USA* 98(5): 2814–19.

Cho RJ, Campbell MJ, Winzeler EA, Steinmetz L, Conway A, Wodicka L, Wolfsberg TG, Gabrielian AE, Landsman D, Lockhart DJ, and Davis RW (1998). A genome-wide transcriptional analysis of the mitotic cell cycle. *Molecular Cell* 2: 65–73.

Chu S, DeRisi J, Eisen M, Mulholland J, Botstein D, Brown PO, and Herskowitz I (1998). The transcriptional program of germ cell development in budding yeast. *Science* 282: 699–705.

DeRisi JL, Iyer V, and Brown PO (1997). Exploring the metabolic and genetic control of gene expression on a genomic scale. *Science* 278: 680–6.

Duggan DJ, Bittner M, Chen Y, Meltzer P, and Trent JM (1999). Expression profiling using cDNA microarrays. *Nat Genet* 21: 10–14.

Geschwind DH, Ou J, Easterday MC, Dougherty JD, Jackson RJ, Chen Z, Antoine H, Terskikh A, Weissman IL, Nelson SF, and Kornblum HI (2001). A genetic analysis of neural progenitor differentiation. *Neuron* 29: 325–39.

Iyer VR, Eisen MB, Ross DT, Schuler G, Moore T, Lee JC, Trent JM, Staudt LM, Hudson J Jr, Boguski MS, Lashkari D, Shalon D, Botstein D, and Brown PO (1999). The transcriptional program in the response of human fibroblasts to serum. *Science* 283: 83–7.

Lashkari DA, DeRisi JL, McCusker JH, Namath AF, Gentile C, Hwang SY, Brown PO, and Davis RW (1997). Yeast microarrays for genome-wide parallel genetic and gene expression analysis. *Proc Natl Acad Sci USA* 94: 13057–62.

Loftus SK, Chen Y, Gooden G, Ryan JF, Birznieks G, Hilliard M, Baxevanis AD, Bittner M, Meltzer P, Trent J, and Pavan W (1999). Informatic selection of a neural crest-melanocyte cDNA set for microarray analysis. *Proc Natl Acad Sci USA* 96: 9277–80.

Luo L, Salunga RC, Guo H, Bittner A, Joy KC, Galindo JE, Xiao H, Rogers KE, Wan JS, Jackson MR, and Erlander MG (1999). Gene expression profiles of laser-captured adjacent neuronal subtypes. *Nat Med* 5: 117–22.

Marshall A and Hodgson J (1998). DNA chips: An array of possibilities. *Nat Biotechnol* 16: 27–31.

Ramsay G (1998). DNA chips: State-of-the-art. *Nat Biotechnol* 16: 40–4.

Rukenstein A, Rydel RE, and Greene LA (1991). Multiple agents rescue PC12 cells from serum-free cell death by translation- and transcription-independent mechanisms. *J Neurosci* 11: 2552–63.

Spellman PT, Sherlock G, Zhang MQ, Iyer VR, Anders K, Eisen MB, Brown PO, Botstein D, and Futcher B (1998). Comprehensive identification of cell-cycle regulated genes in *Saccharomyces cerevisiae*. *Mol Biol Cell* 95: 14863–8.

Wodicka L, Dong H, Mittmann M, Ho M-H, and Lockhart DJ (1997). Genome-wide expression monitoring in *Saccharomyces cerevisiae*. *Nat Biotechnol* 15: 1359–67.

# 7 Oligonucleotide Arrays and Gene Expression Profiling of the Brain: Brainiacs Express Themselves

*Tarif A. Awad, David J. Lockhart, and Carrolee Barlow*

It is sometimes assumed that because the brain is such a complex organ, experimental genomics methods are not directly applicable to neurobiological studies. In fact, it is because the brain and brain processes are complex that it is even more important to apply methods that allow large numbers of genes to be monitored across a significant number of experiments. There are simply too many genes to attack these problems solely in a serial fashion. Given the heterogeneity of the brain, the large numbers of genes encoded in the genomes of higher mammals, and the complexity of processes involved in behavior, learning, and memory, we need to apply the best tools to find the genes that determine important phenotypes and that encode the proteins that carry out specific functions. How can we begin to understand the mechanisms underlying various brain functions, and how can we understand what can and does go wrong in disease? How can such tasks be accomplished without being overly costly and time- and labor-intensive?

Monitoring the expression levels of thousands of genes at a time, for tens or even hundreds of samples, starting with a few micrograms of RNA has, amazingly enough, become somewhat routine with the help of high-density DNA microarrays. We, and others, have put the technology to work to address a variety of biological problems, and in particular to study the brain and various brain functions. This chapter details how to use DNA microarray technology (specifically, Affymetrix oligonucleotide arrays) to determine the genes that are responsible for specific neurological and behavioral phenotypes, the unique activities of different cell types, and the unique structures and functions of different brain regions.

We provide an overview of the technology and examples of specific experiments, paying particular attention to experimental procedures and uses of the technology for neurobiological studies.

### High-Density Oligonucleotide Arrays

The GeneChip platform is an integrated system of genomic tools developed for DNA microarray analysis by Affymetrix, Inc. (Santa Clara, Calif.). The system consists of high-density oligonucleotide probe arrays, instruments for hybridization, washing, and reading of the arrays, and software for data analysis and management. Current applications include highly parallel monitoring of gene expression in several eukaryotes (e.g., human, mouse, rat, yeast, *Drosophila melanogaster*, *Arabidopsis thaliana*) and prokaryotes (*Escherichia coli*), genotyping of human single-nucleotide polymorphisms, and detection of sequence variants in disease-related genes such as p53 (Fodor, 1997; Lipshutz et al., 1995; Lockhart and Winzeler, 2000).

A growing number of published studies and reviews provide a wide perspective on the current uses and possible future applications of oligonucleotide probe array technology. These studies are in fields that include research in cancer and other human diseases (Golub et al., 1999), genotyping and polymorphism analyses (Fan et al., 2000; Mei et al., 2000; Sapolsky and Lipshutz, 1996), drug development (Gray et al., 1998; Kennedy, 2000; Lockhart, 1998), immunology (Der et al., 1998; Glynne et al., 2000), stress response (Jelinsky and Samson, 1999), aging studies (Lee et al., 1999, 2000), neurobiology (Sandberg et al., 2000; Soriano et al., 2000), DNA–protein interactions (Bulyk et al., 1999), and genome-wide functional studies (Cohen et al., 2000; Winzeler et al., 1999).

The heart of the technology is the oligonucleotide probe array, a fingernail-sized glass square with a dense grid of many small physical regions that contain oligonucleotides attached to the surface. The array is encased in a plastic cartridge with a hybridization chamber designed to hold the interrogated sample. Hybridization, staining, and scanning of arrays is largely automated, with instruments controlled by a computer workstation. Gene expression data, whether maintained as individual files or housed in a relational database, is in a highly ordered, consistent format, and can be further analyzed and mined with a variety of both custom and commercial statistical and data visualization and mining tools (e.g., Affymetrix LIMS system, GeneSpring, Spotfire).

### Photolithographic Synthesis of Probe Arrays

Oligonucleotide probe arrays are made by synthesizing large numbers of oligonucleotides *in situ* on a glass surface. The oligonucleotides are synthesized at high density using light-directed, spatially specific combinatorial chemistry (Fodor et al., 1991; McGall et al., 1996). Photolithography, a process used in computer chip manufacturing, uses light that is directed to specific physical locations by a series of masks to etch extremely fine patterns, such as electronic circuits, on wafers layered with conductors and semiconductors.

In the case of DNA probe arrays, light is directed to different regions on an activated glass slide through a series of masks to direct the building of DNA probes with specified sequences (figure 7.1). The oligonucleotide probes are organized into a grid of "probe cells," each cell containing more than a million copies of one spe-

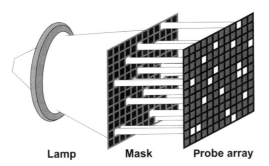

**Lamp**        **Mask**        **Probe array**

**Figure 7.1** Photolithographic synthesis of probe arrays. A cartoon showing a mask used to selectively expose portions of the glass surface to light.

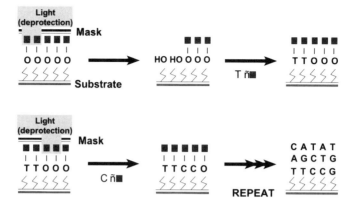

**Figure 7.2** Step-by-step scheme of photolithographic probe array synthesis. Detailed steps in the photolithographic synthesis of probe arrays, showing two cycles of mask exposure followed by the incorporation of a specific nucleoside at designated positions.

cific sequence of DNA. Like computer chips, GeneChip probe arrays begin as wafers (typically 5 × 5 inches square) and are later diced into multiple arrays (49 to 169 or more, depending on the wafer format) that are placed in separate cartridges and used individually.

The chemical synthesis process begins by coating the wafer with a linker that will serve as a covalently bound spacer for the oligonucleotides. A photolabile protecting group (removable with light) prevents the linker from reacting until it is activated. The first mask directs light to preselected probe cells on the wafer. Light removes the protective groups and primes the linker for coupling with a nucleoside (figure 7.2). Other areas on the surface are under the shadow of the mask and are not deprotected. In other words, only the regions that have been irradiated are reactive for the next round of DNA synthesis.

The entire wafer is then bathed with a solution containing the first nucleoside, which is covalently added only at the light-activated areas. The reacting nucleosides are also protected, preventing the repeated incorporation of the nucleoside into the same chain. The process is repeated with each of the subsequent cycles involving the deprotection of specific subsets of probe cells on the wafer with a specific mask, followed by the incorporation of one of the four nucleosides.

The number of steps required to build even hundreds of thousands of different oligonucleotides of a specified length and sequence is less than or equal to $4L$, where $L$ is the length of the longest oligonucleotide on the array. Optimization of mask design reduces the number of synthesis cycles (a 25-mer oligonucleotide array typically requires approximately 80 cycles rather than the theoretical maximum of 100). A reduction in the mask features (i.e., smaller transparent "windows") allows the density of probe cells (and information content per unit area) to be increased without additional synthesis steps.

Currently, Affymetrix produces probe arrays with more than 400,000 different probe cells ($20 \times 20$ μm), each with millions of copies of a specific 25-mer probe. After the synthesis is complete, the wafer is cut into individual arrays that are packaged into plastic cartridges for storage, hybridization, washing, staining, and reading. Parallel synthesis of arrays on wafers produces consistent arrays and allows the quality of different lots of arrays to be checked by test-hybridizing one or two sample arrays from each wafer.

**Design of Arrays for Monitoring Gene Expression**

The high density and uniformity of probe cells on oligonucleotide arrays permit redundancy as well as a variety of controls to be built into the design. In order to increase confidence and improve the accuracy of mRNA quantitation, multiple independent probes (typically 25-mers) are used to detect each expressed sequence (figure 7.3). Each probe is designed to be a "perfect match" (PM) with a specific region of the expressed target sequence. In addition, each PM probe is partnered with a single mismatch (MM) to the target sequence.

The MM probe is synthesized immediately adjacent to its corresponding PM probe, forming a series of PM/MM probe pairs that make up a probe set (figure 7.3) for each gene or expressed se-

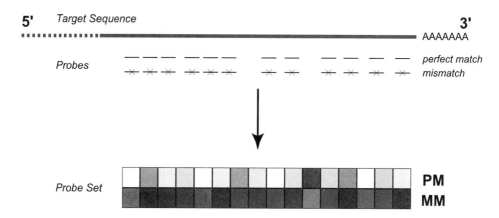

**Figure 7.3** The design of expression probe arrays. The target sequence is used to select multiple unique 25-mer probes, which are synthesized on the array as the perfect match (PM) probes. In addition, control probes, designed with a single mismatch to the target sequence, are synthesized as the mismatch (MM) probes. A group of probes designed to detect one target sequence (or cluster) is called a probe set.

quence tag. The number of probe pairs in each probe set is typically 14 to 20, depending on the type of array. The MM probes in each set provide a measure for nonspecific hybridization, offer a way to determine if the hybridization signal is truly due to the intended messenger RNA, and also provide a convenient way to subtract out the potentially confounding contributions of cross-hybridization and nonspecific background signals.

To design a gene expression array, sequence data are obtained from public sources (such as UniGene) or private databases. Expressed sequences are prepared for probe selection by checking cluster composition and member alignment, then choosing an exemplar or consensus sequence to be used as the target region for probe selection. Probes are chosen starting from the 3′-end of each target sequence and extend, in most cases, up to 600 bases toward the 5′-end. Probe selection for eukaryotes is biased toward the 3′-end to minimize the effects of partial mRNA degradation and incomplete cDNA or cRNA synthesis. Probes are selected according to sequence uniqueness relative to the rest of the genome (and relative to related family members), the absence of expected secondary structure and repeats, and a set of sequence-based selection rules that were derived from theory and empirical observations of oligonucleotide hybridization behavior.

In addition to transcript-specific probe sets, gene expression arrays contain a variety of controls. Some control probes are used to check the quality of the synthesis process, and others provide signals and patterns used for automatic grid alignment and image analysis. In addition, eukaryotic expression arrays contain probe sets for noneukaryotic transcripts (primarily from *E. coli* and *Bacillus subtilis*) that can be "spiked" into the sample to serve as independent controls for the quality of sample preparations and probe array hybridizations. Finally, probe sets representing the 3'- and 5'-ends of several consistently expressed genes (e.g., actin and reduced glyceraldehyde phosphate dehydrogenase [GAPDH] in mammalian cells) in a given species are included. These controls are used to indicate the quality of the input mRNA based on a measurement of the 3' to 5' ratio of the control transcripts. If the 3' to 5' ratio is greater than 2 or 3 for these control genes, the quality of the sample or sample preparation techniques (and therefore the resulting data) may be questionable.

**Sample Preparation and Hybridization**

Total RNA or purified polyA mRNA (in eukaryotes) can be used as starting material for analyzing probe array expression. The RNA sample can be prepared for hybridization in multiple ways (Cho et al., 1998; Lockhart et al., 1996; Warrington et al., 2000; Wodicka et al., 1997), and protocols are constantly being updated and improved (www.affymetrix.com). Since the amount of tissue-specific RNA is sometimes limited, some amplification is useful in order to produce sufficient amounts for hybridization from the least number of cells.

A commonly used protocol requires approximately 200 ng of polyA mRNA or 5–10 μg of total RNA for every sample. Total RNA is actually preferred since it is easier to obtain, fewer cells are needed to give the minimum amount required, and the sample quality is superior. The quality of the cellular RNA is very important for reliable and reproducible results. In general, the 260/280 ratio of the purified input RNA should be as close to 2.0 as possible (1.9–2.1).

The RNA is first used to synthesize double-stranded cDNA that incorporates a T7 promoter sequence at the 3′-end. The resulting cDNA is used as a template in an *in vitro* transcription (IVT) reaction to produce linearly amplified (typically 50- to 200-fold), biotin-labeled, antisense cRNA. The cRNA is randomly fragmented (average length of 30 to 50 bases) and mixed into a hybridization solution that contains hybridization controls and blocking agents.

Hybridization is carried out for 16 hours at 45 to 50 °C in a hybridization oven. The probe arrays are washed and stained using a software-controlled fluidics station. The washing and staining protocol involves using low- and high-stringency washes, followed by a staining step in which a streptavidin–phycoerythrin conjugate is applied to the probe array. The streptavidin–phycoerythrin conjugate binds to the incorporated biotin on the hybridized cRNA, marking it with the fluorescent phycoerythrin. A subsequent antibody amplification step adds additional phycoerythrin molecules, resulting in about a fivefold increase in signal-to-noise ratio. After a final wash, the probe array is ready for scanning. The scanner uses a 488-nm blue argon laser that excites phycoerythrin, and the fluorescence is detected through a 570-nm long-pass filter with confocal optics. The arrays are scanned in about 5 to 10 minutes at a spatial resolution of 3 μm. The signal is digitized (16-bit gray scale) and transferred to a computer workstation for further quantitative image analysis (figure 7.4).

### Analysis of Expression Data

The first data file generated from the signal detection is a large "raw" image file (.DAT file, approximately 45 MB in size for a 1.28 × 1.28-cm array scanned at 3 μm resolution), which is asso-

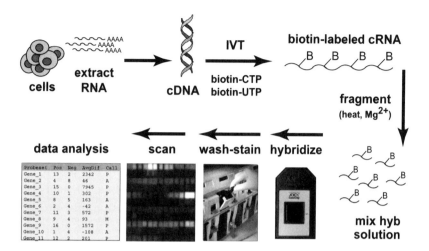

**Figure 7.4**   Sample preparation for expression analysis. In this protocol, double-stranded cDNA is made from the starting RNA; the cDNA is used as a template to make amplified, biotin-labeled cRNA, which is fragmented and hybridized to the array. After washing and staining, the array is scanned.

ciated with user-generated sample and experiment information at the time of the scan. The .DAT file contains pixel-by-pixel data from the probe array scan. Because the pixel size is small, multiple pixels (typically $7 \times 7$) are measured for each probe cell. A signal-averaging algorithm that ignores border pixels and intensity outliers calculates one representative intensity value for every probe cell. The resulting value is saved for each probe cell in the .CEL file (7 to 10 MB in size).

Next, a user-controlled data analysis process is applied to generate qualitative (present/absent, increase/decrease, etc.) and quantitative (relative expression level, fold change) results for every probe set on the array. Probe array analysis can be applied to any single probe array (absolute analysis), or to any pair of arrays of the same type, each hybridized with a different sample (comparison analysis).

The default analysis algorithms examine the data in a number of ways to generate the final qualitative and quantitative results. After background subtraction, normalization or scaling of the data is generally carried out to equalize the overall signal intensities across different arrays used in a given set of experiments.

Next, a number of different metrics are determined for every probe set. For example, each probe pair in a set is checked for specific hybridization performance (PM vs. MM) to ensure reliable detection of the sampled regions of the transcript above the noise of the assay. The various metrics are integrated into a call of "P" for present, "A" for undetected, and "M" for marginal for the transcript or EST cluster represented by the probe set. Because of the use of multiple, independent probes for each gene or EST, it is possible to use a consistent overall pattern of hybridization to the PM and MM probes to determine if the signal is due to the designated transcript.

In effect, the set of probes acts as a jury, with each member given a vote in order to make a qualitative assessment. The members of the jury must agree to a reasonable extent (more like a civil trial in which unanimity is not required) in order to make a call of "present." In this way, no single probe in a set has an undue influence, and this makes the approach much more impervious to the occasional outlier or a strong and unpredictable cross-hybridization event.

In the case of comparison analyses, every probe pair in a set is checked for significant changes in intensity between the two experiments. The software integrates the comparisons for every probe set into a call of "I" for increase, "D" for decrease, and "NC" for no change (along with marginal calls when patterns of change are more ambiguous).

The codified expression algorithms also produce quantitative results that reflect transcript abundance and relative changes between compared samples. The quantitative metric used is termed the *average difference* because it is literally the average of the PM − MM differences across the probes in the set. The average difference for a probe set is calculated as a "trimmed" mean (e.g., after outlier rejection) of the intensity differences (PM minus MM) for each probe pair in the set, and it has the advantage of being automatically background subtracted. The average difference is useful as a measure of expression level because it has a nearly linear relationship with the transcript abundance over a wide dynamic range of more than three orders of magnitude (figure 7.5A).

In addition, an estimate of the relative change, or fold change, of expression levels is calculated based on the ratio of the average difference values between any two experiments (after setting a minimum possible denominator based on the size of the noise to avoid dividing by zero or values that are not significantly above the noise).

### Data Quality and the Importance of Replicates

Oligonucleotide probe arrays, when used correctly, provide consistent, linear quantification of thousands of transcripts in parallel across many samples (figure 7.5). With current methods and standard analysis criteria, mRNAs that are present at a relative abundance of 1:100,000 are readily detected as present, and changes of a factor of 1.8 or greater can be routinely detected with high confidence (1:100,000 corresponds to approximately 1–5 copies per mammalian cell for a pure cell population). A number of factors, however, can contribute to variability and noise in the results. The use of assay controls (such as hybridization spikes), internal sample controls, and other metrics (such as background and noise levels), help determine the quality of a particular array measurement.

When strict procedures are applied during animal and tissue handling, sample preparation, and array hybridization, overall assay variability can be minimized, and the false positive rate can be kept extremely low. For example, we have shown (Sandberg et al., 2000) that the false positive rate in brain mapping studies (as assessed by independently repeating expression measurements on the hippocampus of different mice) was between zero and three genes per ~13,000 measured, while sensitivity to some rare transcripts and small expression changes was maintained (Lockhart and Barlow, 2001b).

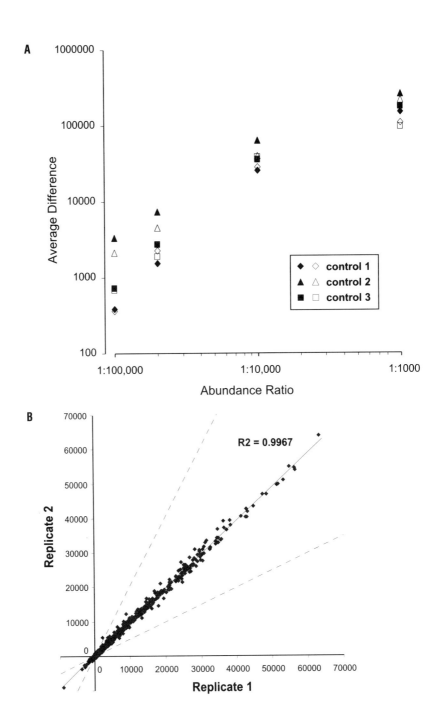

Biological variability is typically greater than assay variability. In general, it is recommended that independent biological replicates be incorporated into the design of any experiment in order to minimize biological (and assay) noise. The number of replicates to use will depend on the intrinsic degree of variability, which can be assessed by a comparison of independently obtained results. The number of independent measurements required for a given level of sensitivity and accuracy needs to be continually assessed based on the consistency of the observations made for the specific type of experiment. If duplicate observations are not sufficiently consistent, then additional replicates need to be performed. The continuous analysis of replicate data, for example, indicates regions, strains, perturbations, or protocols for which the inherent variability is greater, and for these, additional repeats are necessary to maintain the same levels of confidence.

In addition, a larger number of replicates are very useful when attempting to detect and quantify expression differences that are even more subtle than our standard threshold factor of 1.8. As mentioned earlier, if there are expected sources of additional variation (e.g., if genetically identical inbred strains of mice are not used, or for any studies that use human tissue), then a larger number of replicates may need to be performed to ensure the same level of confidence in the results.

One of the advantages of the "single sample per array" approach used with oligonucleotide arrays is that the results for any sample can be compared with those for any other (provided they are hybridized to the same type of probe array). Therefore, variability

**Figure 7.5** Expression assay performance. (*A*) Linearity of the assay is shown with three polyA "spiked" transcripts that are added to the starting mRNA at specified abundance ratios. The measured average difference values for the spikes have a linear relationship with their abundance ratio. (*B*) Reproducibility of the assay is shown with a scatter plot of average difference values from two replicate experiments (log scale). Every point on the graph corresponds to one probe set. Noise is more pronounced at lower signal values, as expected. The dotted diagonal lines correspond to a twofold change.

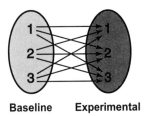

**Baseline      Experimental**

**Figure 7.6**  Pairwise comparisons of replicates. A $3 \times 3$ comparison scheme results in nine comparison files. The reproducibility of quantitative array results allows flexibility in how comparisons are carried out. Comparing all baseline replicates with all experimental replicates and then looking for consistent changes in the resulting comparisons effectively filters out false changes that are due to biological (and assay) variation and noise.

within replicates in a group can be determined as a measure of assay and biological noise within the group.

In addition, comparisons between two groups can be "multiplied," pairing every member of one group with every member of the second group. Using two controls and two experimentals, for example, allows four comparisons. As the number of replicates increases, the number of possible comparisons grows geometrically: $3 \times 3 = 9$, and so on (figure 7.6). Changes in mRNA abundance (increase or decrease calls) that are seen consistently across multiple comparisons of biologically independent replicates are generally of the highest confidence, since experimental noise and intrinsic variation (both biological and assay) are largely filtered out.

## Gene Expression Profiling and Complex Brain Functions

In this section we demonstrate the feasibility of applying advanced genomics methods to studies of the brain and highlight issues that are important for the proper use of the technology. Some aspects of the need for special care were described above—for example, the importance of using inbred strains whenever possible to decrease the "noise" caused by variation in genetic background, and the necessity of employing systematic protocols for dissection and preparation of tissue, RNA, and hybridization samples. Independent verification of array-based results and appropriate nonarray follow-up studies are also discussed.

## Brain Region-Specific Expression Measurements

Determining which genes are expressed and where they are expressed within the brain will help us address a host of interesting questions and will also help to develop new tools. For example, we would like to know which genes are responsible for the unique structures and functions of specific brain regions and the unique processes that are carried out in a region-specific fashion. There is a paucity of site-specific tools in the brain. It is possible that through an analysis of the regulatory elements of uniquely expressed genes, we can identify promoters that can be used to drive the expression of related genes in specific cell types or tissues in animal models.

In order to identify the genes that are responsible for the unique structures and functions of specific brain regions, as well as those that may be responsible for neurobehavioral phenotypes, we measured expression profiles in specific regions of the adult mouse brain (Sandberg et al., 2000). We determined the pattern of gene expression in six different brain regions in two commonly used inbred mouse strains (C57BL/6 and 129SvEv) and in control mouse embryonic fibroblasts. We studied the cortex, cerebellum, midbrain, amygdala, entorhinal cortex, and the hippocampus using the Affymetrix murine subA and subB arrays (which together contain 13,069 probe pairs covering more than 11,000 known genes and ESTs).

In this study, we found that 55% of the genes represented on the arrays were detected as expressed in at least one brain region. The overall expression profiles in different regions of the adult mouse brain are surprisingly similar, but there are a significant number of genes that are differentially expressed between regions. In addition, a small but significant number are uniquely expressed in one region, but not in others (Sandberg et al., 2000; table 7.1; figure 7.7; plate 5). In contrast, 13.6% (1780/13,069) of the monitored genes were differentially expressed between brain tissue and fibroblasts, even though the two very different types of cell populations express a similar overall number of genes. This indicates, as might be expected, that various brain regions are considerably more similar to each other than to fibroblasts.

We have also performed similar experiments on selected brain regions from multiple monkeys and humans (figure 7.7) to test the generality of the observations made in mouse models (Del Rio, Lockhart and Barlow, unpublished). The experiments using human and monkey RNA were performed on the same type of oligonucleotide array that was designed to measure the expression levels of nearly 7000 human genes. Because of the high sequence similarity between most human and monkey genes, monkey experiments can be performed using human arrays without any changes in experimental procedures or major changes in data analysis methods.

The general picture concerning the number of genes that are uniquely expressed and the regions that have the most distinct expression profiles is quite consistent between humans and mice. We compared the specificity profile for homologous human and monkey genes that showed region specificity in the mouse, and we find that many of the genes have similar patterns of expression. However, for many genes the expression patterns are not the same across all three mammals. It is intriguing to speculate that some of these differences give rise to the significant differences in brain function and cognitive abilities between our distantly related cousins and us.

### Gene Expression and Complex Behaviors

A primary goal of neurogenetics is to determine the genes that are responsible for specific neurological and behavioral phenotypes. Fortunately, we can take advantage of the many different inbred

**Table 7.1** Gene expression differences between mouse brain regions

| C57BL/6 (2/2) | Cb | Cx | EC | Hp | Mb | MEF |
|---|---|---|---|---|---|---|
| Ag | 438 | 52 | 28 | 58 | 144 | 2078 |
| Cb | | 333 | 412 | 329 | 242 | 2159 |
| Cx | | | 25 | 27 | 75 | 2070 |
| EC | | | | 63 | 176 | 2115 |
| Hp | | | | | 95 | 2081 |
| Mb | | | | | | 2084 |
| **129SvEv (2/2)** | Cb | Cx | EC | Hp | Mb | MEF |
| Ag | 413 | 46 | 23 | 65 | 154 | 2146 |
| Cb | | 305 | 405 | 368 | 260 | 2137 |
| Cx | | | 20 | 44 | 105 | 2135 |
| EC | | | | 69 | 193 | 2043 |
| Hp | | | | | 149 | 2123 |
| Mb | | | | | | 2136 |
| **C57BL/6 and 129SvEv (3/4)** | Cb | Cx | EC | Hp | Mb | MEF |
| Ag | 470 | 48 | 22 | 70 | 171 | 2261 |
| Cb | | 355 | 439 | 388 | 279 | 2196 |
| Cx | | | 25 | 40 | 118 | 2156 |
| EC | | | | 80 | 232 | 2237 |
| Hp | | | | | 156 | 2258 |
| Mb | | | | | | 2205 |

The number of genes differentially expressed between amygdala (Ag), cerebellum (Cb), cortex (Cx), entorhinal cortex (EC), hippocampus (Hp), midbrain (Mb) and mouse embryonic fibroblasts (MEF). The numbers are based on consistent observations in independent replicates (2/2 for each strain individually or 3/4 for the combined analysis) using the criteria of a 1.8 fold change or greater, a qualitative call of increased, marginally increased, decreased or marginally decreased, a signal change of 50 and a call of present in at least one of the samples, using Affymetrix GeneChip software. (Reproduced with permission, *Nature Reviews Neuroscience*, Lockhart and Barlow, 2001.)

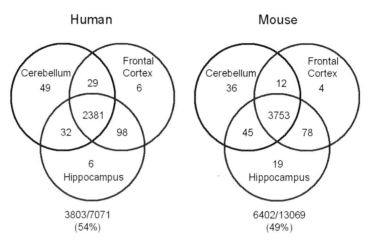

**Figure 7.7**  Of mouse and man. Venn diagrams showing the number of genes with specific expression patterns in a subset of adult human and mouse brain regions. To identify genes with region-restricted expression, genes were classified as "present" in a region if the gene had a call of "present" in at least three out of four samples. Similarly, to classify genes as clearly not detected, we used a call of "absent" in four out of four brain regions (absent or expression at levels below the threshold of detection). The total number interrogated and the number and percentage of genes that scored as present in at least one of the three brain regions is indicated below the diagrams. Note that a higher percentage of genes are observed to be uniquely expressed in human than in mouse cerebellum and frontal cortex. This may be because only portions of these regions were used from human brain whereas the entire structure was used from the smaller mouse brain. (Reproduced with permission from Lockhart and Barlow, 2001a.) See plate 5 for color version.

mouse strains with characterized phenotypes that already exist. These inbred mice are very useful for neurogenetics studies because they have known differences in interesting behaviors, brain anatomy, and sensitivity to environmental perturbations—but in the context of a preexisting and well-defined genetic background.

We used gene expression profiling of multiple brain regions in two commonly used inbred strains (C57BL/6 and 129SvEv) to find genes that might account for the known differences in neurobehavioral phenotypes (Sandberg et al., 2000). Of the more than 7000 genes that are detected in some region of the brain, only 24 were differentially expressed in all six brain regions between the two strains (figure 7.8). An additional 49 genes were differentially expressed between the strains in at least one brain region. This indicates that the expression levels between the strains are quite similar for more than 99% of the genes, and that fewer than 1% determine the differences in phenotype. However, it is important to remember that only about 10,000 genes were on the array (representing about one-third of the genes in the mouse genome), and that only about 60% gave signals in most experiments. That means that by extrapolation to the entire genome, more than 350 genes are probably differentially expressed between the strains in at least one region, which certainly could account for a great deal of the phenotypic variation between these strains.

These results suggest that the combination of global differential expression analysis with traditional mapping and positional cloning approaches may be an efficient route to the identification of disease genes or quantitative trait loci (QTL). The goal is similar for both approaches—to find the genes responsible for complex traits—but in QTL analysis, the genes are identified positionally throughout the genome (Risch, 2000), whereas in expression mapping, genes are identified functionally, based on measurements of gene expression behavior. For example, we found that several differentially expressed genes are encoded in chromosomal regions thought to harbor genes important for strain differences in CNS phenotypes.

In particular, *GIRK3* (more highly expressed in 129SvEv) is located on chromosome 1 in a region that has been shown to contain one or more of the genes that contribute to strain differences for free running period and locomotor activity (Mayeda and Hofstetter, 1999), aspects of fear-conditioned response (cued and contextual) (Caldarone et al., 1997; Wehner et al., 1997), open-field emotionality (Flint et al., 1995), and acute pentobarbital-induced seizures (Buck et al., 1999). *GIRK3* plays a role in maintaining resting potential and in controlling the excitability of the cell (Kubo et al., 1993) and should be considered a candidate for involvement in modulating multiple CNS phenotypes.

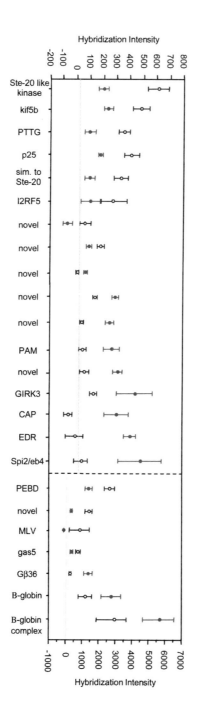

The two approaches are complementary in that standard QTL analysis identifies the genes (or loci) that harbor genetic differences relevant to a phenotype, while the expression approach measures cellular consequences of the variation. Although conventional QTL analysis is powerful for mapping susceptibility loci to chromosomal intervals, many genes usually reside in these large intervals, and extensive additional work is required to identify the specific gene or genes involved. An expression-based strategy may be useful for identifying candidate genes while simultaneously identifying additional genes that may act to modify the particular trait being studied.

### Verification and Follow-up of Array-Based Observations

Although the array-based expression measurements can be made highly quantitative and reproducible, specific genes that are found to be differentially expressed on arrays should be viewed as high-probability candidates. Based on our experience and that of others, the importance of great experimental care, well-characterized and rigorous analysis, and the need for appropriate follow-up and verification cannot be overemphasized.

In almost all cases, when verifying candidates and designing experiments, experiments should be performed *at least* in duplicate, with replicates performed as *independently* as possible (e.g., different mice or independent dissections of a region, independent

**Figure 7.8**  Gene expression differences between C57BL/6 and 129SvEv mouse strains. Shown are the hybridization signals of the 24 genes differentially expressed in all brain regions in C57BL/6 and 129SvEv mouse strains. Each gene is represented by a mean value based on the hybridization intensity from the 12 individual samples for each strain (six brain regions in duplicate) (open circles represent C57BL/6 and filled circles 129SvEv). The y-axis is labeled with hybridization intensities ranging from $-200$ to 800 (left side of graph) and $-1000$ to 7000 (right side of graph), separated by a hatched vertical line. The horizontal line indicates the noise level. Error bars represent the 95% confidence interval derived from the 12 values for the six different brain regions for each strain. (Reproduced with permission from Sandberg et al., 2000.)

sample preparations, and independent hybridizations to physically different arrays). It is not sufficient to merely remake samples from the same RNA extracted from the same mouse or tissue sample, or to simply rehybridize samples to additional arrays. If genetically identical inbred mice are not used, then it is necessary to perform additional experiments or to pool mice to effectively average out differences that are due to genetic heterogeneity (independently pooled samples should be used as replicates). The same considerations apply when using any other animal or human tissue.

We routinely use Northern blotting and quantitative RT-PCR for selected sets of genes to verify results and to validate experimental and analytical methods. In these follow-up experiments, it is important to use independently prepared samples and *not* simply the same RNA that was used for the array experiments (for an example, see figure 7.9). Independent verification is even more critical if untested or less stringent analysis criteria are used, or if extremely subtle expression differences are to be interpreted. In addition, Western blots can be used to measure corresponding protein levels, and immunohistochemistry and *in situ* hybridization can be used to measure cell or region specificity of proteins and mRNAs. These techniques can be very useful in both confirming and extending the results obtained using mRNA measurements on arrays.

Finally, global expression measurements should be considered as a starting point for gaining understanding of a biological problem, and as a valuable tool for obtaining information concerning a large number of genes. These methods should be used in the context of other types of measurements, knowledge, and information, and it should be understood that findings will often need to be followed up with further experiments of various, more conventional types.

## Summary

We have provided an overview of the use of DNA array gene expression technology for the study of the brain and complex brain

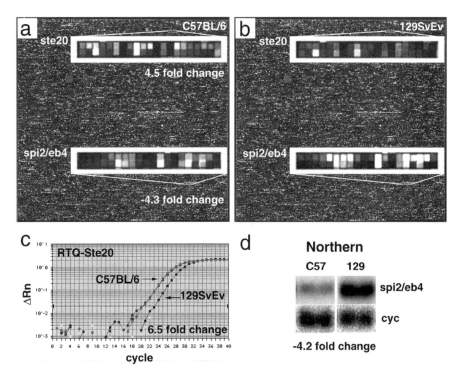

**Figure 7.9** Array results and follow-up analysis. Array images following hybridization of RNA from the hippocampus of a C57BL/6 and a 129SvEv mouse. The array shown covers more than 6000 murine genes and ESTs. The expanded images show the raw data for the probe sets for two genes (ste20 and spi2/eb4) found to be differentially expressed in the two strains, along with the magnitude of the expression changes. The array results were confirmed using quantitative RT-PCR (Taqman) and Northern blots. The expression results for these genes are in qualitative and quantitative agreement for the different methods; for ste20, the array indicated a 4.5-fold and RT-PCR a 6.5-fold change; for spi2/eb4, the array indicated a change of $-4.3$-fold, while the Northern blot results indicated a $-4.2$-fold change. (Reproduced with permission from Lockhart and Barlow, 2001b.)

functions. This field may be considered to be in its infancy and many new developments are expected. Clearly, we need more complete gene coverage, more information about variant splice forms of genes, and improved methods for amplification and analysis of small amounts of RNA. In addition, because the datasets are so large and the amount of information so great, it is important to consider how best to use and understand data on this scale, how to distribute them, and how to present them, since conventional journal articles and Excel spreadsheets or large text files are insufficient.

What new types of bioinformatics tools need to be developed to interrogate the data, to make sense of the complex relationships between genes, and to make the data broadly available and accessible to the entire scientific community? It is clear that gene expression profiling allows us to move beyond conventional one-gene-at-a-time approaches to those that look broadly at the activity of tens of thousands of genes in parallel. As such, it provides a foundation for asking system-level questions.

The careful, rigorous, systematic, creative, and innovative uses of these genomics tools are opening up new avenues for the study of the brain, and allowing questions to be addressed in ways that would have been completely impractical only a few years ago. There is no doubt that the advances in gene targeting technology, robust behavioral analysis, and global gene expression measurements will provide new approaches to the study of the brain and further our ability to understand the interplay between the genes that give rise to complex behaviors and unique brain functions.

## Acknowledgments
We would like to thank Cindy Doane, Jo A. Del Rio, Todd A. Carter, Daniel G. Pankratz, Lisa Wodicka, Edward Callaway, and members of the Barlow laboratory for their advice and assistance.

# References

Buck K, Metten P, Belknap J, and Crabbe J (1999). Quantitative trait loci affecting risk for pentobarbital withdrawal map near alcohol withdrawal loci on mouse chromosomes 1, 4, and 11. *Mamm Genome* 10: 431–7.

Bulyk ML, Gentalen E, Lockhart DJ, and Church GM (1999). Quantifying DNA–protein interactions by double-stranded DNA arrays. *Nat Biotechnol* 17: 573–7.

Caldarone B, Saavedra C, Tartaglia K, Wehner JM, Dudek BC, and Flaherty L (1997). Quantitative trait loci analysis affecting contextual conditioning in mice. *Nat Genet* 17: 335–7.

Cho RJ, Fromont-Racine M, Wodicka L, Feierbach B, Stearns T, Legrain P, Lockhart DJ, and Davis RW (1998). Parallel analysis of genetic selections using whole genome oligonucleotide arrays. *Proc Natl Acad Sci USA* 95: 3752–7.

Cohen BA, Mitra RD, Hughes JD, and Church GM (2000). A computational analysis of whole-genome expression data reveals chromosomal domains of gene expression. *Nat Genet* 26: 183–6.

Der SD, Zhou A, Williams BR, and Silverman RH (1998). Identification of genes differentially regulated by interferon alpha, beta, or gamma using oligonucleotide arrays. *Proc Natl Acad Sci USA* 95: 15623–8.

Fan J-B, Chen X, Halushka MK, Berno A, Huang X, Ryder T, Lipshutz RJ, Lockhart DJ, and Chakravarti A (2000). Parallel genotyping of human SNPs using generic oligonucleotide tag arrays. *Genome Res* 10(6): 853–60.

Flint J, Corley R, DeFries JC, Fulker DW, Gray JA, Miller S, and Collins AC (1995). A simple genetic basis for a complex psychological trait in laboratory mice. *Science* 269: 1432–5.

Fodor S (1997). Massively parallel genomics. *Science* 277: 393–4.

Fodor SPA, Read JL, Pirrung MC, Stryer L, Lu AT, and Solas D (1991). Light-directed, spatially addressable parallel chemical synthesis. *Science* 251: 767–73.

Glynne R, Akkaraju S, Healy JI, Rayner J, Goodnow CC, and Mack DH (2000). How self-tolerance and the immunosuppressive drug FK506 prevent B-cell mitogenesis. *Nature* 403: 672–6.

Golub TR, Slonim DK, Tamayo P, Huard C, Gaasenbeek M, Mesirov JP, Coller H, Loh ML, Downing JR, Caligiuri MA, Bloomfield CD, and Lander ES (1999). Molecular classification of cancer: Class discovery and class prediction by gene expression monitoring. *Science* 286: 531–7.

Gray NS, Wodicka L, Thunnissen AM, Norman TC, Kwon S, Espinoza FH, Morgan DO, Barnes G, LeClerc S, Meijer L, Kim SH, Lockhart DJ, and Schultz PG (1998). Exploiting chemical libraries, structure, and genomics in the search for kinase inhibitors. *Science* 281: 533–8.

Jelinsky SA and Samson LD (1999). Global response of *Saccharomyces cerevisiae* to an alkylating agent. *Proc Natl Acad Sci USA* 96: 1486–91.

Kennedy GC (2000). The impact of genomics on therapeutic drug development. *Exs* 89: 1–10.

Kubo Y, Baldwin T, Jan Y, and Jan L (1993). Primary structure and functional expression of a mouse inward rectifier potassium channel. *Nature* 362: 127–33.

Lee CK, Klopp RG, Weindruch R, and Prolla TA (1999). Gene expression profile of aging and its retardation by caloric restriction. *Science* 285: 1390–3.

Lee CK, Weindruch R, and Prolla TA (2000). Gene-expression profile of the aging brain in mice. *Nat Genet* 25: 294–7.

Lipshutz RJ, Morris D, Chee M, Hubbell E, Kozal MJ, Shah N, Shen N, Yang R, and Fodor SP (1995). Using oligonucleotide probe arrays to access genetic diversity. *Biotechniques* 19: 442–7.

Lockhart DJ (1998). Mutant yeast on drugs. *Nat Med* 4: 1235–6.

Lockhart DJ and Barlow C (2001a). Expressing what's on your mind. *Nat Rev Neurosci* 2(1): 63–8.

Lockhart DJ and Barlow C (2001b). Methods in neurogenetics. In *DNA Arrays and Gene Expression Analysis in the Brain*, S Moldin and H Chin, eds. CRC Press, Boca Raton, Fla., pp. 143–70.

Lockhart DJ and Winzeler EA (2000). Genomics, gene expression and DNA arrays. *Nature* 405: 827–36.

Lockhart DJ, Dong H, Byrne MC, Follettie KT, Gallo MV, Chee MS, Mittmann M, Wang C, Kobayashi M, Horton H, and Brown EL (1996). Expression monitoring by hybridization to high-density oligonucleotide arrays. *Nat Biotechnol* 14: 1675–80.

Mayeda AR and Hofstetter JR (1999). A QTL for the genetic variance in free-running period and level of locomotor activity between inbred strains of mice. *Behav Genet* 29: 171–6.

McGall G, Labadie J, Brock P, Wallraff G, Nguyen T, and Hinsberg W (1996). Light-directed synthesis of high-density oligonucleotide arrays using semiconductor photoresists. *Proc Natl Acad Sci USA* 93: 13555–60.

Mei R, Galipeau PC, Prass C, Berno A, Ghandour G, Patil N, Wolff RK, Chee MS, Reid BJ, and Lockhart DJ (2000). Genome-wide detection of allelic imbalance using human SNPs and high density DNA arrays. *Genome Res* 10(8): 1126–37.

Risch NJ (2000). Searching for genetic determinants in the new millennium. *Nature* 405: 847–56.

Sandberg R, Yasuda R, Pankratz DG, Carter TA, Del Rio JA, Wodicka L, Mayford M, Lockhart DJ, and Barlow C (2000). From the cover: Regional and strain-specific gene expression mapping in the adult mouse brain. *Proc Natl Acad Sci USA* 97: 11038–43.

Sapolsky RJ and Lipshutz RJ (1996). Mapping genomic library clones using oligonucleotide arrays. *Genomics* 33: 445–56.

Soriano MA, Tessier M, Certa U, and Gill R (2000). Parallel gene expression monitoring using oligonucleotide probe arrays of multiple transcripts with an animal model of focal ischemia. *J Cereb Blood Flow Metab* 20: 1045–55.

Warrington JA, Nair A, Mahadevappa M, and Tsyganskaya M (2000). Comparison of human adult and fetal expression and identification of 535 housekeeping/maintenance genes. *Physiol Genomics* 2: 143–7.

Wehner JM, Radcliffe RA, Rosmann ST, Christensen SC, Rasmussen DL, Fulker DW, and Wiles M (1997). Quantitative trait locus analysis of contextual fear conditioning in mice. *Nat Genet* 17: 331–4.

Winzeler E, Lee B, McCusker J, and Davis R (1999). Whole genome genetic-typing in yeast using high-density oligonucleotide arrays. *Parasitology* 118(Suppl): S73–80.

Wodicka L, Dong H, Mittmann M, Ho M-H, and Lockhart DJ (1997). Genome-wide expression monitoring in *Saccharomyces cerevisiae*. *Nat Biotechnol* 15: 1359–67.

## 8 The Use of Fixed Human Postmortem Brain Tissue to Study mRNA Expression in Neurodegenerative Diseases: Applications of Microdissection and mRNA Amplification

*Vivianna M. D. Van Deerlin, Stephen D. Ginsberg, Virginia M.-Y. Lee, and John Q. Trojanowski*

Great progress has been made toward understanding the underlying molecular pathophysiology of many neurodegenerative disorders. However, there are still myriad unanswered questions about the mechanisms of neurodegeneration. Genetic material preserved by fixation in human postmortem brain tissue is an excellent resource for addressing some of these questions because whereas fresh or frozen tissue is frequently not available, archives of fixed human tissue exist in many institutions. New molecular techniques now make it possible to isolate and study both genomic DNA and total RNA from fixed paraffin-embedded tissue (PET) (von Weizsacker et al., 1991; Shibata et al., 1991; Crisan and Mattson, 1993; Stanta and Schneider, 1991; Mizuno et al., 1998; Gall et al., 1993).

As new genes linked to neurodegenerative disorders are discovered, it is possible to search retrospectively for mutations in the genomic DNA of tissue from patients with a neurodegenerative disease. Similarly, the profile of messenger RNA in the brain tissue of such patients provides a real-time snapshot of the state of gene expression in the tissue prior to fixation.

However, the brain is a complex structure with heterogeneous neuronal and nonneuronal cellular populations. Each distinct cell type is likely to have a unique pattern of gene expression or "molecular fingerprint" under normal and pathological conditions. Furthermore, differences in gene expression may also exist even within a single class of cells. Thus, the pattern of mRNA expression in a subpopulation of cells or single cells is more likely to be informative than the pattern in a whole-tissue homogenate. Indeed, the molecular underpinnings of why certain neuronal cell populations are vulnerable to neurodegeneration, often termed "selective vulnerability," may be elucidated by single-cell mRNA analyses more readily than by utilizing regional and total brain preparations.

Isolation of small homogeneous cell populations or single cells from tissue can be accomplished using techniques for microdissection. The mRNA from one or a few cells can be amplified in a linear fashion with a technique called "antisense amplified RNA" (Kacharmina et al., 1999; Phillips and Eberwine, 1996; Crino et al., 1996; Eberwine et al., 1992b; Van Gelder et al., 1990). Thus, mRNAs directly isolated or amplified from normal and diseased tissue can be used to study the differential gene expression pattern of single candidate genes by a variety of methods, including reverse-transcriptase polymerase chain reaction amplification, or multiple genes simultaneously using expression array analysis. Indeed, studies of well-preserved mRNA in archived brain tissue with emerging technologies for the recovery and amplification of mRNA for gene expression analysis are likely to open the door to new discoveries in the normal and diseased human nervous system.

## RNA from Fixed Human Tissue

The analysis of fixed tissue is of interest to the study of neurodegenerative diseases because the bulk of archived human brain tissue is fixed and of postmortem origin. While many institutions have their own sources of autopsy brain tissue, there are also several brain banks with archived tissue (Colantuoni et al., 2000).

Although surgical biopsies or resections are useful, their availability for use in research studies is limited in most institutions. Cell lines may serve as excellent research model systems, but they have limitations and cannot completely replace human tissue for the study of gene expression in the pathogenesis of human disease. Therefore, much effort has been focused on optimizing the use of DNA and RNA in fixed tissue for research on human diseases.

Standard methods of DNA analysis from formalin-fixed paraffin-embedded tissue, such as Southern hybridization, have historically been impeded by partial degradation of the DNA resulting from the fixation process (Crisan and Mattson, 1993). The advent of DNA amplification by the polymerase chain reaction permitted the use of archived fixed tissue for retrospective analyses of DNA, despite partial degradation, by specifically targeting small regions for amplification (Shibata et al., 1991; Crisan and Mattson, 1993; Gall et al., 1993; Crisan et al., 1990). Not long after the successful analysis of DNA from formalin-fixed PET tissue, success with RNA analysis in PET was reported (von Weizsacker et al., 1991; Stanta and Schneider, 1991; Jackson et al., 1990, 1989; Finke et al., 1993). Although RNA is known to be much less stable than DNA and extremely susceptible to degradation by intrinsic and environmental ribonucleases, RNA is sufficiently preserved in some fixed tissues to allow for Northern analysis and RT-PCR amplification (Stanta and Schneider, 1991; Mizuno et al., 1998).

The implication of these technological advances in nucleic acid analysis was that archived tissue blocks, representing a vast and invaluable source of information, were no longer useful just for their histology or immunohistochemical properties. Archived tissue blocks were now also valuable for their DNA and RNA content, which could be used to probe genomic DNA for mutations or specific sequence variations and to detect the presence and/or levels of mRNAs for analysis of gene expression.

By modifying standard RNA extraction methods, RNA can be isolated from PET (Coombs et al., 1999; Goldsworthy et al., 1999; Masuda et al., 1999; Krafft et al., 1997). Further modifications allow the use of these methods for isolation of RNA from small numbers of cells microdissected from PET (Goldsworthy et al., 1999). In addition to published protocols (Mizuno et al., 1998; Finke et al., 1993; Coombs et al., 1999; Masuda et al., 1999; Foss et al., 1994), there are also now several commercially available kits for isolation of RNA from PET (Ambion, Austin, Texas; Zymo Research, Orange, Calif.).

When working with RNA from single or very few cells, the RNA is usually not extracted by these methods, but rather may be amplified using antisense RNA amplification (Kacharmina et al., 1999;

Phillips and Eberwine, 1996; Crino et al., 1996; Eberwine et al., 1992b; Van Gelder et al., 1990). Some investigators have reported direct RT-PCR amplification in single cells (Rappolee et al., 1989; Chiang, 1998; Glowatzki, 1997; Glowatzki et al., 1995; Tong et al., 1994; Hu et al., 1997). Alternatively, mRNA levels can be examined *in situ* either by *in situ* hybridization (ISH) (Kadkol et al., 1999), *in situ* RT-PCR (Zhou et al., 2000; Muratori, 1998; Thaker, 1999), or *in situ* transcription (IST) (Eberwine et al., 1992a; Tecott et al., 1988). These methods are often complementary to one another and which one is used depends on the question being asked. Frequently more than one method is necessary to confirm an observed difference in gene expression (Crino et al., 1998; Ginsberg et al., 1999a; Hemby et al., 2002).

The quality of RNA in fixed tissue, for example its relative integrity, is variable from tissue block to tissue block. However, by what criteria does one judge "RNA quality"? RNA of quality acceptable for one downstream application may not be of sufficient quality for another and vice versa. For example, failure to amplify RNA by RT-PCR in one PET block may not affect the block's utility for methods such as IST. Furthermore, RNA does not need to be intact to be detected. Whereas methods such as ISH give little indication of the integrity of the RNA, especially when short riboprobes are used, if RNA degradation has occurred, Northern hybridization analysis will reveal a smear rather than a band of the appropriate size for a full-length transcript (Morrison-Bogorad et al., 1995; Ross et al., 1992; Barton et al., 1993). Finally, the level of degradation or integrity of RNA at the whole-tissue level does not indicate its state at the single-cell level.

These confounding factors may lead one to ask the question: Is "RNA quality" in fixed tissue really important? The answer may depend on whether the research study is prospective or retrospective. In a prospective study, the investigator has the choice of preparing the tissue optimally for the intended application, making RNA quality a priority. However, in a retrospective study using archived tissue, often there is not a great deal of choice of tissue blocks, especially when studying uncommon diseases. In this scenario, investigators must do their best to utilize and study the available tissue. In either case, an understanding of how the RNA is affected by processing can help interpret the experimental results.

There are many factors that may affect the quality of the RNA in fixed tissue, including the amount of time before fixation (i.e., the postmortem interval or PMI for autopsy-derived tissue), antemortem clinical variables such as agonal state, tissue pH, patient medications, the choice of fixative, the length of time in fixative before processing, and the time the tissue is stored after fixation. Many investigators have examined these critical factors in an effort to optimize the analysis of RNA from fixed tissue.

## Antemortem and Postmortem Effects on RNA Stability

All postmortem brain tissue is not the same, even if the clinical or pathological diagnosis is the same. Essential differences include the PMI, the agonal state of the patient prior to death, the patient's drug regimen, and presumably other less well-defined factors. The PMI and agonal state are known to affect neurochemical measures (Barton et al., 1993; Kontur et al., 1994). Although analysis of RNA is possible under many circumstances, even when partial degradation has taken place, the state of RNA preservation in postmortem tissue may be important for subsequent analysis. Although most studies examining the stability of RNA postmortem have been done on frozen tissue using ISH (Kingsbury et al., 1995), Northern hybridization (Morrison-Bogorad et al., 1995; Ross et al., 1992; Kingsbury et al., 1995; Johnson et al., 1986; Leonard et al., 1993), or RT-PCR (Schramm et al., 1999; Johnston et al., 1997), it is reasonable to infer that similar effects on RNA stability would be observed in fixed tissue, although fixation has its own additional effects on RNA stability.

Antemortem variables arise from alterations in the physiological state of the individual at the time of death. In several studies, agonal state has been shown to influence the stability of mRNA in brain tissue (Barton et al., 1993; Kingsbury et al., 1995; Johnston et al., 1997). Kingsbury et al. (1995) found that tissue pH correlated strongly with preservation of four mRNA species in three brain areas by ISH and Northern blot hybridization. These authors speculate that postmortem tissue pH may serve as a measure of the patient's antemortem state of hypoxia, with lower pH assumed to result from prolonged hypoxia, thereby leading to decreased stability of the mRNA, independent of the underlying disease process. Other investigators have reached similar conclusions (Johnston et al., 1997). Therefore, pH may serve as a rough measure of RNA stability, but since a great deal of scatter exists in the pH values, no absolute pH cutoff value can guarantee that the RNA is well preserved.

It is also important to note that antemortem variables may affect the stability of different mRNA species to varying degrees. For example, one group found that antemortem fever increases the level of hsp 70 mRNAs in Alzheimer's disease (AD) brain (Morrison-Bogorad et al., 1995; Barton et al., 1993). Amyloid precursor protein (APP) mRNA levels are increased by hypoxia and fever; seizures affect a variety of transcripts; and thyroid hormone influences the splicing pattern of the microtubule-associated protein tau (Barton et al., 1993).

The PMI, the amount of time that elapses between the time of death and the denaturation or freezing of a tissue sample, is considered to be a major postmortem variable. It is interesting, however, that the length of the PMI, even up to 84 hours, has been shown to have no significant effect on RNA stability with regard to parameters such as quantity of extractable RNA, quantity of poly(A)$^+$ mRNA, specific mRNAs, and intactness of RNA (Mizuno et al., 1998; Barton et al., 1993; Kingsbury et al., 1995; Johnson et al., 1986; Leonard et al., 1993; Schramm et al., 1999; Perrett et al., 1998). However, selective degradation of certain mRNA species postmortem, for example hsp 70, has been documented (Barton et al., 1993; Pardue et al., 1994). Therefore, before studying a specific transcript extensively in postmortem tissue, it may be important to show that PMI does not affect its level dramatically.

Both antemortem and postmortem influences can affect the levels and stability of all mRNAs or some mRNA species selectively. These variables may change the apparent gene expression profile of cells independent of the disease process, which could introduce artifacts. As an example, failure to take agonal effects into account could lead one to the wrong conclusion because apparent differences in gene expression between diseased and control brains may be incorrectly ascribed to the disease process, when in fact the difference is an antemortem phenomenon. Antemortem influences such as agonal state do not invalidate the analysis of mRNA from postmortem samples, but they do need to be considered in the design of the experiment and the interpretation of results.

## Effects of Fixation and Storage on RNA Quality

Fixation is used to denature and preserve tissue; however, the process has a profound effect on the molecular properties of nucleic acids and proteins. Fixatives generally function by either creating crosslinks and thereby altering the structure and function of macromolecules (e.g., aldehyde derivatives such as formalin) or by exerting a precipitative effect (e.g., ethanol). Optimal preservation of tissue morphology for histological examination must be balanced against the need for preservation of nucleic acids for analysis. Factors that can affect the quality of RNA in the fixed tissue include the chemical composition of the fixative, the duration of fixation, and the amount of time the tissue is stored in paraffin blocks.

## Choice of Fixative

There are numerous choices of fixatives for tissue preservation; they commonly include 10% neutral-buffered formalin (NBF), 4% paraformaldehyde, and 70% ethanol. Many studies have examined the effect of the chemical composition of the fixative on the utility of the fixed tissue for downstream applications involving RNA analysis (Goldsworthy et al., 1999; Koopmans et al., 1993; Foss et al., 1994; Tournier et al., 1987; Weiss and Chen, 1991). Amplification of mRNA by RT-PCR from PET was more frequently successful when either ethanol, acetone, or OmniFix II, an alcohol-based fixative (Zymed Laboratories, South San Francisco, Calif.), were used as the tissue fixative, while results with formalin have been mixed (Ben-Ezra et al., 1991; Koopmans et al., 1993; Foss et al., 1994).

In general, fixatives containing mercuric chloride and/or potassium dichromate, such as B-5 and Zenker's, have more deleterious effects on nucleic acid isolation than milder fixatives such as formalin because mercury and chromium have a high affinity for protein side chains, leading to large metal–protein complexes that are relatively resistant to digestion and disaggregation (Crisan and Mattson, 1993; Ben-Ezra et al., 1991; Greer et al., 1991a). Acid fixatives such as those containing picric acid, acetic acid (Carnoy's), and Bouin's solution are also generally not compatible with subsequent nucleic acid analysis (Greer et al., 1991a; Ben-Ezra et al., 1991; Foss et al., 1994). Experience in our laboratory with acridine orange (AO) histofluorescence, a fluorescent dye that intercalates into nucleic acids, and aRNA amplification methodologies indicate that brain tissues fixed in NBF and 70% ethanol with 150 mM sodium chloride work optimally, whereas tissues fixed in Bouin's solution yield poor results (Ginsberg et al., 1999a, 1997, 1998).

The introduction of novel methods for the assessment of gene expression in single cells poses unique challenges for optimal tissue fixation. For example, Goldsworthy and colleagues (1999) compared the effects of different fixatives on tissue morphology, ease of microdissection by laser capture, and RNA integrity as determined by RT-PCR amplification. The following fixatives were compared on both frozen and paraffin-embedded mouse liver tissue: 70% ethanol, 95% ethanol, 10% NBF, and 3% paraformaldehyde. In addition, acetone and Rapid-Fixx (75% methanol, 20% formaldehyde, 5% glacial acetic acid; Shandon, Pittsburgh, Pa.) were used for frozen tissue and PLP fixative (2% paraformaldehyde, 7.5 mM L-lysine, and 10 mM sodium periodate) on PET (Goldsworthy et al., 1999).

The fixatives were compared for their morphological quality, completeness of microdissection, and quantity of mRNA, as assessed by RT-PCR amplification of either $\beta_2$-microglobulin or glyceraldehyde-3-phosphate dehydrogenase (Goldsworthy et al., 1999). The precipitative fixatives ethanol and acetone consistently produced more RT-PCR amplification product than formalin, although overall more amplification product was obtained from frozen tissue than from PET. However, amplification of mRNA from PET was only successful when a small ($\sim$80-base) sequence was targeted and a sensitive quantitative amplification method, TaqMan real-time RT-PCR analysis (PE Biosystems, Foster City, Calif.), was used. The use of 70% ethanol also produced good morphologic quality and tissue quality for microdissection. For PET, the PLP fixative also gave good results by the same criteria (Goldsworthy et al., 1999).

If amplification by RT-PCR were the only criterion by which to judge mRNA quality, then ethanol would appear to be the fixative of choice. However, for examination of cellular mRNA by ISH, fixation with either 10% NBF or 4% paraformaldehyde consistently appears to give the best results, as judged by reproducibility and intensity (Kadkol et al., 1999; Tournier et al., 1987; Weiss and Chen, 1991). Therefore, the fixation protocol should be chosen with forethought about downstream applications. Frequently more than one method is applied to confirm results of gene expression analysis, such as RT-PCR and ISH. With this in mind, the use of more than one fixative should be considered when rare or irreplaceable tissue is procured. While appropriate in RT-PCR, formalin-fixed tissue does not work well for array hybridizations and frozen or ethanol-fixed tissue is preferred (Karsten et al., 2002).

**Duration of Fixation**

Increased duration of fixation has a negative effect on the subsequent analysis of mRNA by virtually all methods. In most cases only relatively short target sequences, up to $\sim$270 bases, can be amplified by RT-PCR from formalin-fixed PET (Mizuno et al., 1998; Goldsworthy et al., 1999; Krafft et al., 1997; Koopmans et al., 1993; Foss et al., 1994; Stanta and Bonin, 1998). Increased fixation time (more than 18 hours) decreases the size of the targets that can be amplified (Greer et al., 1991b; Masuda et al., 1999). The reason for this size limitation has traditionally been ascribed to either degradation of the RNA before or during fixation or the cross-linking effects of the fixative. However, chemical modification of the RNA by formalin, e.g., hydroxymethylation and methylene bridge formation, has also been considered (Crisan and Mattson, 1993).

The chemical modification of RNA by formalin and its effect on amplification by RT-PCR was studied by Masuda et al. (1999). In order to examine the effect of increased fixation time on the length of mRNA target that could be amplified by RT-PCR from formalin-fixed mouse liver tissue, they designed 16 primer pairs that targeted either the apolipoprotein E, apolipoprotein A, or $\beta_2$-microglobulin genes. The primer pairs were designed to yield a ladder of RT-PCR product sizes ranging from 135 to 4035 base pairs.

Their results showed that an increased fixation time of between 16 hours and 7 days decreased the maximal size of RT-PCR product amplified. This decrease in maximal target size was not due to degradation of the RNA because the total RNA as determined by gel electrophoresis was intact. To show that chemical modification was a factor, the RNA was heated for 1 hour at 70 °C in Tris-EDTA buffer in an attempt to demodify the RNA. This demodification treatment increased the maximal length of the amplified product that could be obtained by RT-PCR compared with analysis of RNA from fresh tissue. This effect was more prominent in the tissue that was fixed for a shorter time.

Masuda and colleagues (1999) studied the chemical modification of RNA further by in vitro fixation of synthetic ribonucleotide oligomers followed by time-of-flight mass spectroscopy analysis. The results were consistent with the addition of monomethyl groups and methylene bridge formation between bases. These effects were greatest on adenines and cytosines, both of which have a free amino group. This is of special interest with regard to methods that make use of the poly(A)$^+$ tail of mRNA for priming reverse transcription, such as RT-PCR and IST.

These results suggest that chemical modifications may be at least in part responsible for the inability to amplify long fragments by RT-PCR from RNA in fixed tissue. Some of these modifications may be reversed by manipulations such as heating extracted RNA species to 70 °C, or digestion with proteinase K (Masuda et al., 1999). With prolonged incubation in formalin, however, the chemical modifications may become irreversible. These results do not rule out the possibility that prolonged fixation may also partially degrade RNA. Additional work to confirm the fixation-induced chemical modifications of RNA and to improve methods to reverse or ameliorate these modifications is warranted.

Investigators wishing to perform RNA analysis from PET should be aware of the possible influences that fixation could have on the tissue being studied. If RT-PCR experiments are performed, they should be designed, whenever possible, to minimize the effects of fixation by choosing small target fragments for amplification or by using random primers to reverse transcribe the RNA.

### Length of Storage

Extended freezer storage of postmortem tissue has been shown to result in decreased stability of RNA (Leonard et al., 1993; Johnston et al., 1997). Leonard and colleagues (1993) found that storage of human postmortem brain at 70 °C for more than 5 years may compromise its use for oligo(dT)-primed library construction and in vitro expression studies. However, these authors concluded that enough full-length or partial-length mRNA remained after storage to allow RT-PCR amplification, although they recommended priming with random primers rather than with oligo(deoxythymidine) [oligo(dT)] to avoid reliance on the stability of the poly(A)$^+$ tail, which may be more susceptible to modification or degradation (Leonard et al., 1993).

After fixation and paraffin embedding of a tissue sample, the length of time the paraffin block containing the fixed tissue is stored prior to analysis is also important for RNA stability. In general, blocks more than a few years old have decreased amplification efficiency, although RNA has been successfully amplified by RT-PCR from blocks as old as 79 years (Mizuno et al., 1998; Coombs et al., 1999; Krafft, 1997). The main factor determining success of amplification in older blocks was choosing primers that produce a small fragment size, for example, less than 150 bases, by PCR amplification (Krafft et al., 1997).

## Microdissection

Analysis of gene expression in complex tissues, such as the nervous system, is best done in conjunction with a microdissection technique to address changes that occur within distinct populations of cells individually. Neurodegenerative diseases are frequently focal or only involve one or a few cell types, and within the nervous system, the major classes of distinct cells include neurons, macrophages, astrocytes, oligodendroglia, and meningothelial and vascular cells. Neuronal populations are further categorized based upon their morphology, chemical phenotype, and regional/laminar/ nuclear localization (e.g., neocortical pyramidal neurons, hippocampal interneurons, hypothalamic paraventricular nucleus, magnocellular neurons).

If the disease of interest involves only one of these cell types, and that cell type comprises only a small percentage of the total cells in a brain region of interest (e.g., gray matter containing neurons and glial and vascular cells), then analysis of gene expression using a homogenate of this region will be overrepresented by the gene expression pattern of the most common cell type and underrepresented by a less abundant class of cells.

An alternative approach is the analysis of single cells, but this strategy may be complicated by the fact that not all cells of a single class are identical or equally affected by a particular disease process. For example, neurofibrillary tangle (NFT) pathology in AD brain does not affect every neuronal cell type to the same degree, and variability in the deposition and accumulation of NFTs as well as senile plaques (SPs) is found within individual AD patients.

In addition to regional and laminar variation of NFT/SP formation, vulnerable cell types such as hippocampal CA1 pyramidal cells do not display identical pathology because some cells bear prominent NFTs, whereas adjacent cells appear devoid of, or contain few, paired helical filaments of hyperphosphorylated tau (PHFtau), the proteinaceous building blocks of NFTs (West et al., 1994; Hyman et al., 1984; Ginsberg et al., 1999b; Braak and Braak, 1991). Furthermore, analysis of a single cell may not be fully representative of the disease process (which is a dynamic cascade of events that may progress over many years) owing to differences in gene expression among individual cells of the same class, even in a small well-defined brain region. As a result, approaches to studying gene expression in microdissected cellular subpopulations require either analysis of multiple combined cells or multiple individual analyses of single cells (Hemby et al., 2002; Ginsberg et al., 2000). The number of cells needed for the latter approach to achieve statistical significance is not known, but this will depend undoubtedly on the reproducibility of the gene expression patterns generated from studies of similar cells.

Messenger RNA analysis at the single-cell level can be accomplished in situ by ISH or in situ RT-PCR or by amplification of mRNA from microdissected cells (Kacharmina et al., 1999; Phillips and Eberwine, 1996; Crino et al., 1996; Eberwine et al., 1992b; Van Gelder et al., 1990; Kadkol et al., 1999; Zhou et al., 2000; Thaker, 1999; Ginsberg et al., 1999a; Luo et al., 1999; Ghasemzadeh et al., 1996; Cheetham et al., 1997). Microdissection under microscopic visualization has become a very important technique for the analysis of gene expression in a few or single cells. The advantage of microdissection over ISH is that microdissection affords much more flexibility in terms of the methods for the analysis of gene expression and the number of genes studied simultaneously (Kacharmina et al., 1999).

The tissue used for microdissection can be stained or unstained to identify cells of interest. Most often, immunohistochemical labeling of tissue is used to identify individual neurons or other cells on the basis of specific protein expression, which may be associated with a disease process. For example, antibodies directed against hyperphosphorylated tau and amyloid-$\beta$ peptides have been used to identify NFTs and SPs for single-cell aRNA analyses (Ginsberg et al., 1999a, 2000). TUNEL staining has also been used to identify apoptotic cells (O'Dell et al., 1998).

If stained tissue will be used for subsequent mRNA analysis, the staining procedure must be done under ribonuclease-free conditions and the effect of the staining method on the mRNA must be ascertained; for example, some stains are known to inhibit subsequent PCR amplification (Burton et al., 1998). In addition, histochemical stains that indicate the presence of nucleic acids such as AO histofluorescence can be employed to identify tissue specimens from individual cases with suitable RNA preservation (Ginsberg et al., 1997, 1998).

Several methods have been developed to microdissect tissue sections. In one method, ablation is used to destroy or remove the unwanted cells, thereby leaving the area of interest available for subsequent mechanical isolation. Alternatively, a clean, pointed, sharp tool such as a needle, blade, or pulled glass pipette can be used under microscopic visualization to microdissect the tissue or cells of interest manually or with the aid of a micromanipulator (Cheetham et al., 1997; Zhuang et al., 1995; Phillips and Eberwine, 1996).

A commercially available kit called the Pinpoint Slide RNA Isolation System (Zymo Research, Orange, Calif.) allows cells to be isolated in a targeted area of tissue 1–20 mm$^2$ in size. The kit involves placing a solution on the area of interest and allowing it to dry. As the solution dries, the underlying cells become embedded within the dried solution and the area can then be easily microdissected, lifted, and transferred to a tube for RNA extraction. Although this method simplifies microdissection of small regions, it is not meant for isolation of single cells.

Single cells can be isolated using a micropipette combined with a micromanipulator (figures 8.1 and 8.2). Similar micropipettes are

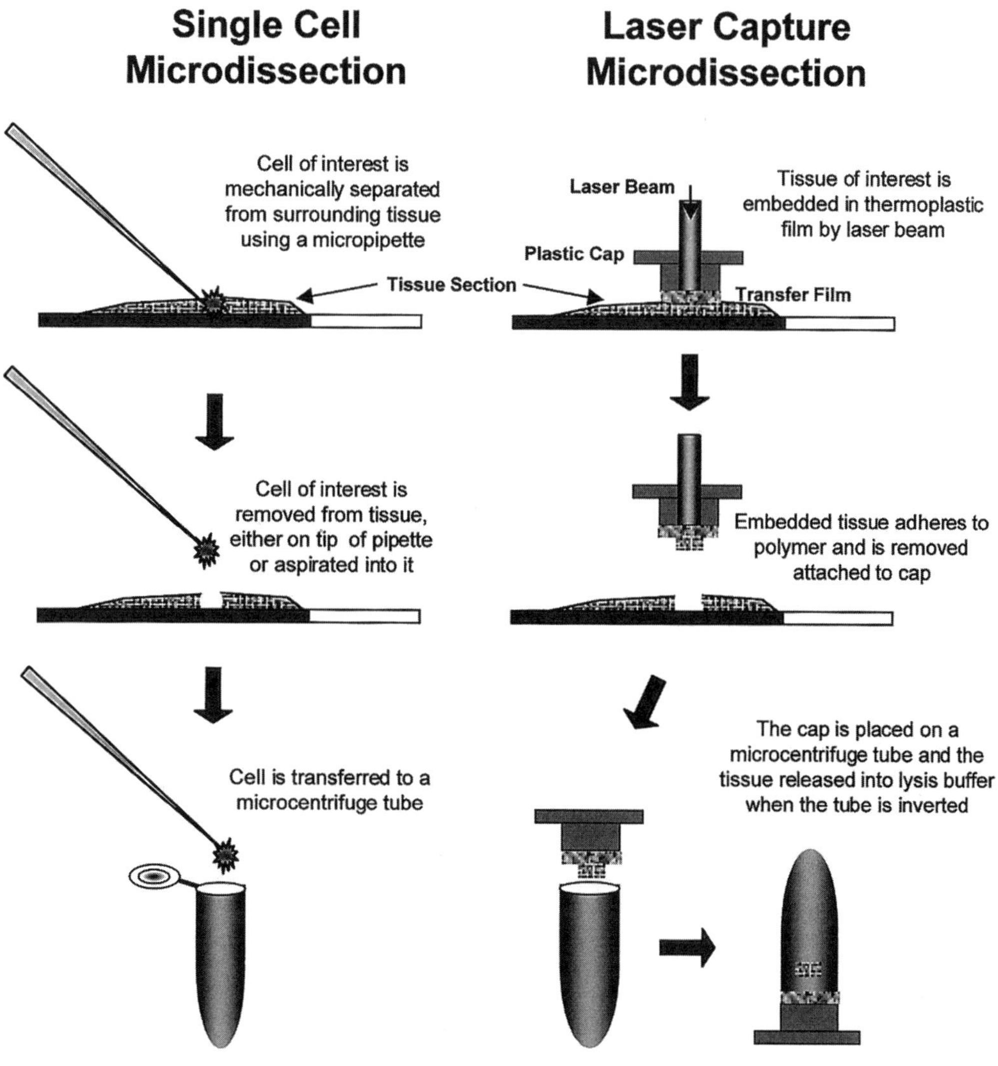

**Figure 8.1** Comparison of single-cell microdissection with laser capture microdissection. Single cells can be microdissected with a micropipette under direct visual guidance using a micromanipulator. The cell can be physically attached to the tip of the micropipette (as shown in this schematic) or aspirated into the fluid-filled pipette. Laser capture microdissection can also be used to isolate one or more cells from paraffin-embedded tissue.

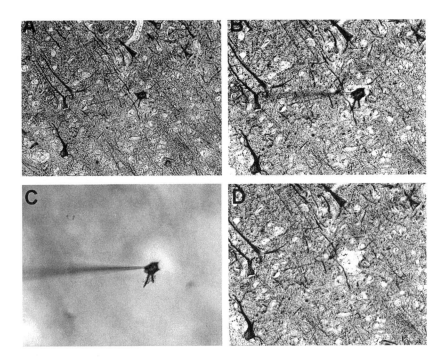

**Figure 8.2** Single-cell microdissection. (*A*) Large pyramidal neurons from an ethanol-fixed paraffin-embedded human brain cortex are shown stained with the neurofilament antibody, RMdO20 (100×). The stained sections are covered with a thin layer of water (rather than a glass cover slip) to facilitate the identification and retrieval of the labeled cell of interest. (*B*) The tip of an Eppendorf Femtotip micropipette (Hamburg, Germany) is shown physically separating the central neuron from the surrounding neuropil (200×). (*C*) The microdissected neuron is attached to the tip of the micropipette and lifted above the plane of the glass slide (200×). (*D*) Tissue section after microdissection and removal of the labeled single neuron of interest (200×).

used routinely in electrophysiological analyses. In fact, when the tissue of interest is living, electrophysiological measurements can be combined with analysis of mRNA (Eberwine et al., 1992b; Van Gelder et al., 1990). Micropipettes can either be homemade using a micropipette puller (for example, from Sutter Instrument Co., Novato, Calif.) or purchased, for example, Femtotips (Eppendorf, Hamburg, Germany). Single cells from PET and fixed frozen sections can be aspirated into the pipette chamber if the diameter of the tip is sufficiently wide, or the cell can be speared by the pipette tip for removal (figure 8.2). In either case, the microdissected cell is transferred into a microcentrifuge tube for subsequent analysis (figure 8.1), but this method requires some degree of manual dexterity and patience.

Laser capture microdissection has also become a reliable and popular method for microdissection of small regions of tissue sections (Bonner et al., 1997; Simone et al., 1998). This method requires a special LCM instrument (Arcturus Engineering, Mountain View, Calif.) that uses a pulsed laser beam to focally bond cells of interest to a transfer film placed directly above the cells. The film is then removed with the cells bound to it (figure 8.1). If desired, this process can be repeated with additional cells. One advantage of the LCM technique is that the morphology of the microdissected cells is preserved. Originally, the diameter of the laser dissecting beam was 30 μm, allowing microdissection of only very large single cells. A modification of the original LCM instrument has been developed that allows the microdissection of smaller-sized single cells (Suarez-Quian et al., 1999). There is no evidence that the laser damages the integrity of the nucleic acids (Suarez-Quian et al., 1999).

## Linear Amplification of RNA

The quantity of RNA in a single microdissected cell, which is estimated to be between 0.1 and 1.0 pg, is not sufficient to allow for standard RNA extraction (Kacharmina et al., 1999; Phillips and

Eberwine, 1996). Therefore, alternative methods of analysis have been used. Specific mRNA transcripts in a single cell can be localized and even roughly quantitated by ISH in multiple cells simultaneously with a riboprobe specific to the transcript of interest (Kadkol et al., 1999; Chow et al., 1998). Alternatively, individual gene transcripts may be amplified directly in single cells by RT-PCR (Hu et al., 1997; Rappolee et al., 1989; Chiang, 1998; Glowatzki, 1997; Glowatzki et al., 1995; Tong et al., 1994). This method has the disadvantage that following the initial cDNA synthesis step by reverse transcriptase, the subsequent amplification by PCR is exponential. Unless careful quantitative RT-PCR is performed, the PCR step of the amplification can induce a great deal of variation from cell to cell—as much as fivefold in one study (Brail et al., 1999). In addition, to attain the necessary level of sensitivity, often the PCR step uses a second round of amplification with nested primers that are internal to the initial set. The disadvantage of this approach is the high risk of contamination when using nested primers and the small number of genes that can be analyzed simultaneously.

In contrast, aRNA involves linear amplification of the mRNA using T7 RNA polymerase so that direct quantitation of the relative abundances of different mRNA species in the single cell can be determined (Kacharmina et al., 1999; Phillips and Eberwine, 1996; Crino et al., 1996; Eberwine et al., 1992b; Van Gelder et al., 1990). The resultant amplified aRNA has been shown to maintain a proportional representation of the starting mRNA (Van Gelder et al., 1990). The aRNA amplification procedure can be applied to a variety of sources, including immunohistochemically identified neurons, NFTs, and SPs (Crino et al., 1996; Ginsberg et al., 1999a, 2000; Cheetham et al., 1997). Each round of aRNA amplification results in approximately a thousandfold amplification, so that after two rounds, a millionfold amplification may be obtained (Kacharmina et al., 1999).

The schematics of the aRNA amplification procedure are shown in figures 8.3 and 8.4. The first step in aRNA amplification

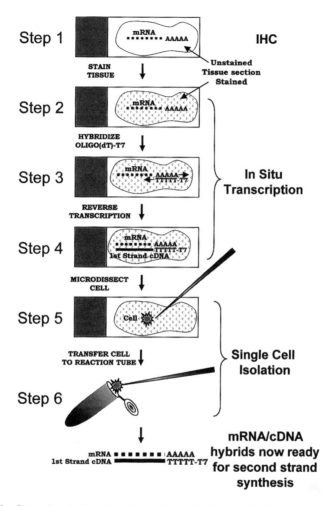

**Figure 8.3** Steps in single-cell isolation for mRNA amplification. The presence of poly(A)$^+$ mRNA in the cells of a tissue section is indicated by the dashed line in step 1. At the microdissection step, a cell is shown instead of the mRNA schematic (step 5). At the end of steps 1–6 the tube contains an mRNA-cDNA hybrid that is ready for second-strand synthesis.

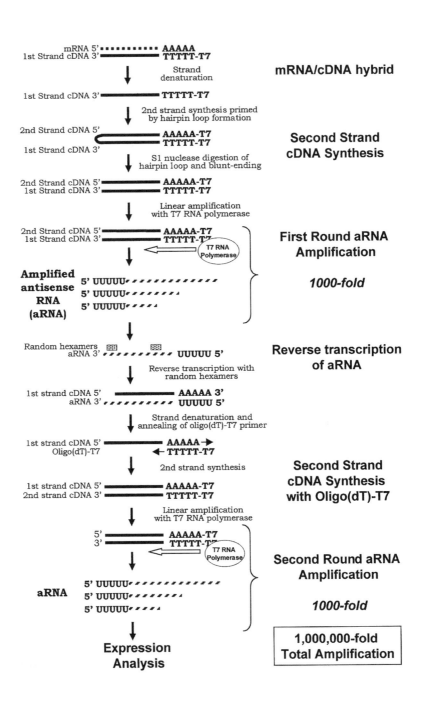

mRNA 5' ▪▪▪▪▪▪▪▪▪▪▪ AAAAA
1st Strand cDNA 3' ━━━━━━━ TTTTT-T7

↓ Strand
denaturation

**mRNA/cDNA hybrid**

1st Strand cDNA 3' ━━━━━━━ TTTTT-T7

↓ 2nd strand synthesis primed
by hairpin loop formation

2nd Strand cDNA 5' ━━━━━━━ AAAAA-T7
━━━━━━━ TTTTT-T7
1st Strand cDNA 3'

**Second Strand
cDNA Synthesis**

↓ S1 nuclease digestion of
hairpin loop and blunt-ending

2nd Strand cDNA 5' ━━━━━━━ AAAAA-T7
1st Strand cDNA 3' ━━━━━━━ TTTTT-T7

↓ Linear amplification
with T7 RNA polymerase

2nd Strand cDNA 5' ━━━━━━━ AAAAA-T7
1st Strand cDNA 3' ━━━━━━━ TTTTT-T7
T7 RNA Polymerase

**First Round aRNA
Amplification**

**Amplified
antisense
RNA
(aRNA)**
5' UUUUU ╱╱╱╱╱╱╱╱╱╱╱
5' UUUUU ╱╱╱╱╱╱╱
5' UUUUU ╱╱╱╱

*1000-fold*

↓

Random hexamers ▦    ▦ ╱╱╱ UUUUU 5'
aRNA 3' ╱╱╱╱╱╱╱╱╱

**Reverse transcription
of aRNA**

↓ Reverse transcription with
random hexamers

1st strand cDNA 5' ━━━━━━━ AAAAA 3'
aRNA 3' ╱╱╱╱╱╱╱╱╱ UUUUU 5'

↓ Strand denaturation and
annealing of oligo(dT)-T7 primer

1st strand cDNA 5' ━━━━━━━ AAAAA →
Oligo(dT)-T7 ← TTTTT-T7

↓ 2nd strand synthesis

1st strand cDNA 5' ━━━━━━━ AAAAA-T7
2nd strand cDNA 3' ━━━━━━━ TTTTT-T7

**Second Strand
cDNA Synthesis
with Oligo(dT)-T7**

↓ Linear amplification
with T7 RNA polymerase

5' ━━━━━━━ AAAAA-T7
3' ━━━━━━━ TTTTT-T7
T7 RNA Polymerase

↓

**aRNA**
5' UUUUU ╱╱╱╱╱╱╱╱╱╱╱
5' UUUUU ╱╱╱╱╱╱╱
5' UUUUU ╱╱╱╱

**Second Round aRNA
Amplification**

*1000-fold*

↓

**Expression
Analysis**

**1,000,000-fold
Total Amplification**

is hybridization of a 66-nucleotide oligo(dT) primer with a 5' attached bacteriophage T7 RNA polymerase promoter binding site [oligo(dT)$_{24}$-T7] to the endogenous poly(A)$^+$ mRNA directly in the tissue section (figure 8.3). Synthesis of cDNA is initiated *in situ* by reverse transcription of the mRNA with avian myeloblastosis reverse transcriptase (AMV-RT; Seikagaku America, Falmouth, Mass.) (Houts et al., 1979). Thus, after this IST step, each newly synthesized cDNA strand will have an incorporated T7 RNA polymerase promoter site.

Cells of interest are selected for the expression of a specific protein marker by immunohistochemical staining prior to hybridization of the oligo and cDNA syntheses (figure 8.3). With the aid of a micromanipulator under microscopic visualization, single cells can be aspirated and placed in a microcentrifuge tube. The reverse transcription step with oligo(dT)$_{24}$-T7 is repeated on the isolated cell as a precautionary measure. The cDNA is dissociated from the mRNA by heat denaturation and then made double stranded by hairpin-loop second-strand synthesis using a Klenow fragment of *Escherichia coli* DNA polymerase I and T4 DNA polymerase (figure 8.4). S1 nuclease is used to cleave the hairpin loop, and the double-stranded cDNA is blunt ended with the Klenow fragment.

The blunt-ended, double-stranded cDNA is now ready for *in vitro* transcription by the T7 RNA polymerase, which recognizes the double-stranded promoter-binding site. The orientation of the promoter is such that the transcribed RNA is antisense to the poly-(A)$^+$ RNA. The result of the transcription is a linear amplification of all the cDNA species in the original sample. To achieve higher levels of aRNA amplification, a second round of aRNA amplifica-

**Figure 8.4** Steps in antisense mRNA amplification. Messenger RNA is indicated by a dashed line; cDNA is indicated by a solid line; and amplified antisense RNA is indicated by the diagonally striped line. T7 indicates the promoter sequence to which the T7 RNA polymerase binds in double-stranded DNA to initiate transcription of aRNA. At the end of two rounds of mRNA amplification, an approximately $1 \times 10^6$-fold linear amplification of the starting mRNA has occurred. The final aRNA product can be used as a probe for expression analysis.

tion can be performed. During the second round of linear aRNA amplification, a radiolabeled nucleotide can be incorporated and the resulting aRNA product can be used as a probe for expression analysis by reverse Northern blot or cDNA microarrays. The aRNA method is reviewed in several references (Kacharmina et al., 1999; Phillips and Eberwine, 1996; Ginsberg et al., 1999b).

The aRNA product, when radiolabeled and analyzed by denaturing gel electrophoresis, has a broad size distribution ranging from a few hundred bases to 4.4 kb, indicating that at least some large cDNAs are synthesized (Cheetham et al., 1997; Ginsberg et al., 1999a). However, not all mRNA species are amplified. Using aRNA products amplified from PET to screen a cDNA library, positivity was identified for only ~15% of the clones, whereas values of 50–75% have been reported for aRNA amplification of single live neurons (Crino et al., 1996). What this means in practical terms is that false negatives may be more of a concern than false positives. This is because a gene shown to be differentially expressed between two cell populations can be confirmed by alternative testing, such as ISH, whereas a false negative will simply not be identified. Again, awareness of the technique's limitations is the key scientific principle.

Another limitation of the technique to be aware of is that owing to the amplification procedure, the aRNA products are generally not full length and are biased toward the 3′-end of the transcript because of priming with an oligo(dT) in the first RT step (Phillips and Eberwine, 1996; Crino et al., 1996). However, since this bias is the same for all the amplified mRNAs, the relative levels can be compared (Madison and Robinson, 1998). When choosing cDNAs for expression analysis, it is important to select clones that contain representation of the 3′-end of the transcript. Another option is to assess multiple ESTs or partial cDNAs or oligonucleotides linked to the same gene. This approach is feasible when employing high-density microarrays with the capability of arraying hundreds or thousands of features. For example, we have assessed the relative expression of the tyrosine kinase domain and the extracellular domain for the high-affinity nerve growth factor receptors trkA, trkB, and trkC in single neurons from normal and AD brains (Ginsberg et al., 2000, 1999a).

The aRNA amplification procedure has been performed on isolated fixed or live cells. If single live cells are studied, the aRNA studies can be combined with studies of electrophysiological parameters (Kacharmina et al., 1999). For analysis of fixed cells, fixation in ethanol appears to be optimal, although an extensive comparison for this technique has not been performed (Kacharmina et al., 1999). Tissue can be fixed and paraffin embedded or fixed immediately after frozen sectioning. When fixed tissue is used for aRNA amplification, several controls should be performed. Confirmation that the PET block selected for analysis has intact total RNA can be done by AO histofluorescence, which stains all RNA species, but does not differentiate mRNA (Ginsberg et al., 1997, 1998).

Alternatively IST, the first step of aRNA amplification, can be performed using a radiolabeled ribonucleotide in the presence and absence of reverse transcriptase enzyme (Tecott et al., 1988). The *in situ* transcribed sections can then be examined by autoradiography after extensive washing, looking for a greater signal from the enzyme-containing reaction than the no-RT control. The mRNA-cDNA hybrids from the IST step (nonradiolabeled) can also be extracted from the entire section and an aliquot then amplified according to the aRNA procedure. Finally, after the IST step, several no-cell controls, tubes into which no cell is placed, should be processed alongside the aRNA tubes containing single cells to control for contamination during the protocol.

## Gene Expression Analysis

The combination of microdissection and aRNA amplification provides a powerful technology that can be used to probe diverse developmental and neurodegenerative disease processes that affect the brain by quantitative analysis of mRNA species. The mRNA from one cell or multiple pooled cells can be amplified in a linear fashion to produce amplified antisense mRNA. There are at least two main avenues that expression analysis can take (figure 8.5).

The first of these is the expression analysis of candidate genes hypothesized and/or known to be involved in disease pathogenesis. Methods applied in this approach include gene-specific RT-PCR, nuclease protection assays, ISH, gene-specific IST, or custom cDNA macroarrays. The latter are sometimes referred to as "reverse Northern blots" because the cDNA "probe" is bound to a nylon membrane in either a dot or slot-blot format and the unknown, labeled RNA sample is then hybridized to the membrane (Phillips and Eberwine, 1996; Crino et al., 1996; Ginsberg et al., 1999a, 2000; Cheetham et al., 1997).

The second expression analysis approach is often referred to as "expression profiling," and is usually a large-scale approach aimed at the simultaneous analysis and comparison of many genes. Expression profiling of many known and unknown genes has been made possible by the extensive information database being generated by the genome and expressed sequence tag sequencing projects. Knowledge of the expression profile of a tissue, cellular subpopulation, or even a single cell will most certainly play an essential role in the functional characterization of known and newly identified genes and the determination of their role in the pathophysiology of diseases. Platforms that assess expression of a large number of cDNA or EST sequences include cDNA microarrays, large-scale cDNA macroarrays on nylon membranes, and oligonucleotide expression arrays (Gene Chip, Affymetrix Inc., Santa Clara, Calif.) (Lockhart et al., 1996; Duggan et al., 1999; Lipshutz et al., 1999; Brown and Botstein, 1999).

**Candidate Gene Approach to Expression Analysis**

Expression analysis using amplified aRNA enables detection of the presence of mRNA species and quantitative assessment of the relative expression levels of multiple mRNAs expressed in

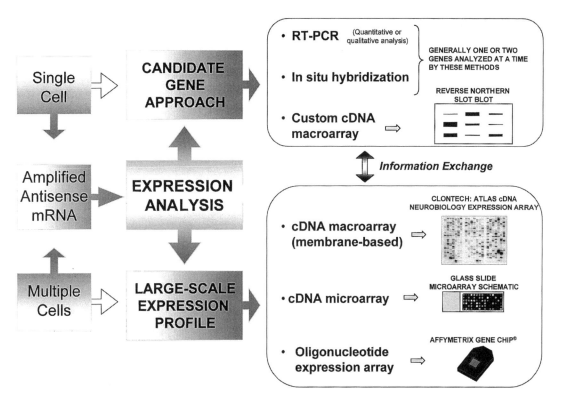

**Figure 8.5** Approaches to expression analysis. A schematic of a reverse Northern blot is shown, with the intensity of the band corresponding to the expression level of the gene represented by the relative intensity of each slot. Large-scale expression profiling by cDNA macroarrays (e.g., macroarrays available from Clontech), cDNA microarrays (e.g., homemade or commercially available glass slide cDNA arrays), or oligonucleotide expression arrays available from Affymetrix (Santa Clara, Calif.), have been used for expression analysis of RNA from various sources. A membrane-based macroarray with 488 neurobiology-related and control genes (Clontech, Palo Alto, Calif.) hybridized with $^{32}$P-labeled mRNA from cultured cells is shown as an example. The ultimate goal is to be able to use these expression analysis platforms to assess the relative abundance of transcripts expressed in a single cell or pooled mRNAs from groups of isolated single cells.

immunohistochemically identified isolated cells in fixed sections of postmortem brain. In the candidate gene approach to expression analysis, the amplified aRNA product is used to assess the quantitative or relative expression levels of a limited number of known genes. The amplification of mRNA from individual cells in fixed PET archival human specimens has been applied to understanding the molecular pathophysiology of tuber formation in tuberous sclerosis as well as assessing the mRNA content of single neurons, senile plaques, and neurofibrillary tangles within the AD brain (Crino et al., 1996; Ginsberg et al., 1999a, 2000). In addition, numerous other studies have applied the aRNA amplification technology to assess the expression of selected candidate genes (Ghasemzadeh et al., 1996; Chow et al., 1998; Nair et al., 1998).

The sequestration of abundant RNA in SPs and NFTs of AD is a unique finding among neurodegenerative disease lesions (Ginsberg et al., 1997). Assessment of aberrant mRNA expression in diseased neurons of AD brains is providing remarkable insights into the pathogenesis of SPs and NFTs.

Antisense RNA amplification was used by Ginsberg and colleagues to screen 51 candidate genes implicated in the pathogenesis of plaques and tangles or the degeneration of neurons in AD simultaneously between single immunohistochemically identified SPs in sections of hippocampus from AD brain and CA1 in brains of normal age-matched controls (Ginsberg et al., 1999a). The relative expression levels were determined by reverse Northern (slot-blot) hybridization in conjunction with ISH and RT-PCR. The results of this aRNA study confirmed that multiple mRNA species are found in individual extracellular SPs in AD. Furthermore, the pattern of mRNAs in the SPs aspirated from the AD brain sections was predominantly neuronal, which may imply that SPs sequester the remnants of degenerating and/or dying neurons and their processes as they form (Ginsberg et al., 1999a).

Differences in gene expression between single CA1 neurons from early- and late-stage AD brain have also been studied by aRNA amplification and reverse Northern (dot-blot) hybridization to 20 candidate and control cDNA clones selected on the basis of their potential relevance to the pathogenesis of AD (Chow et al., 1998). Numerous differences, both up- and downregulation, in gene expression were identified. Sophisticated statistical analyses, including analysis of variance (ANOVA) and canonical analysis of the results were used to assess the validity of the conclusions. The relevance of these differences in candidate gene expression to the pathogenesis of AD has yet to be determined (Chow et al., 1998).

### Large-Scale Expression Analysis

In contrast to the candidate gene approach, large-scale expression analysis is amenable to discovery of new genes by permitting simultaneous analysis of a large number of clones. The applicability of microdissection and aRNA amplification to large-scale cDNA microarrays was recently established (Luo et al., 1999). To study differences in gene expression between morphologically distinct small and large neurons of the rat dorsal root ganglion, Luo and colleagues (1999) used LCM to isolate separate sets of 1000 small or large neurons from ethanol-fixed frozen sections followed by two rounds of aRNA amplification.

The aRNA product was hybridized to a glass slide cDNA microarray containing 477 different cDNA probes, most of which were expected to represent genes preferentially expressed in DRGs. Within a particular class of neuronal subtypes, the expression patterns were reproducible in triplicate experiments. Between the two cell types, 40 genes were found to be differentially expressed, and for 12 of these, similar results were verified by ISH studies, although the extent of the relative differences tended to be greater by ISH than by the cDNA microarray (Luo et al., 1999).

The application of aRNA amplified from single cells to cDNA microarrays using fluorescence labels is limited by the sensitivity of detection. However, the use of radiolabeled aRNA probes to hybridize to large-scale membrane-based expression arrays has been reported by Ginsberg and colleagues (2000). The relative abundance of multiple mRNAs in tangle-bearing vs. normal CA1 neurons aspirated from ethanol-fixed hippocampal PETs of AD and normal brain was studied to examine changes in gene expression associated with the formation of NFTs within neurons in AD.

Immunohistochemical staining for PHFtau was used to identify tangle-bearing neurons, while tangle-free neurons were identified with an antibody directed against nonphosphorylated neurofilament proteins. The mRNA in the isolated neurons was amplified by two rounds of linear T7 RNA polymerase-based RNA amplification with incorporation of a $^{33}$P label in the second round of amplification. The amplified aRNAs were hybridized in parallel to a large-scale membrane-based expression array of more than 18,000 genes and ESTs (Incyte Genomics, Palo Alto, Calif.).

Relative to normal CA1 neurons, those harboring NFTs in AD brains showed significant changes in the expression levels of several classes of transcripts, including mRNAs encoding known phosphatases or kinases, cytoskeletal proteins, synaptic proteins, glutamate receptors, and dopamine receptors implicated in AD neuropathology (Ginsberg et al., 2000). In particular, an EST sequence linked to cathepsin D was identified as being significantly upregulated in the AD tangle-bearing neurons.

Many of the observed differences from the large-scale array were confirmed using aRNA probes hybridized to custom-made cDNA/EST macroarrays (reverse Northern slot blots) (Ginsberg et al., 2000). The custom macroarray included 120 cDNA or EST clones, of which 72% had sequence representation on the large-scale arrays, as well as numerous candidate genes involved in AD. A correspondence of 85% was observed between the expression results from the two platforms. Therefore the combination of the large-scale expression array with a custom macroarray provided the basis for new gene discovery, confirmation of results, and analysis of candidate gene expression.

This report is among the first describing large-scale expression analyses of mRNA derived from single cells in normal brains and in brains with neurodegenerative disease. The analysis on a commercial cDNA membrane-based array was made possible by the high degree of sensitivity afforded by the radiolabeled probe. In parallel with mRNA amplification strategies, a number of signal-enhancing methods are being developed so that the amount of total RNA or polyA RNA needed to perform a microarray experiment is decreasing. For example, the Perkin Elmer Life Sciences (NEN) MicroMax cDNA microarrays (Boston, Mass.) incorporate a detection amplification step with tyramide; and novel probes with signal enhancements (3DNA, Genisphere, Oakland, N.J.) have been developed that require only 1–2 µg of total RNA for cDNA microarray hybridization. Undoubtedly, cDNA microarray expression analysis of single cells will soon become commonplace.

Single-cell expression profiling on high-density cDNA microarrays may become technically feasible; however, the caveat to proceed with caution may be appropriate. Determination of a cell's expression profile requires that the mRNA available for analysis from the cell contain a complete representation of the genes being expressed at a given point in time. In the case of an amplified aRNA product, this is probably not the case, especially when the cell was obtained from a fixed tissue section. In single living cells, the best-case scenario, the aRNA population may represent only 75% of the expressed genes, and this value appears to be significantly lower in aRNA from fixed single cells (Kacharmina et al., 1999; Crino et al., 1996). Therefore, a negative result could represent a true negative, that is, no difference in expression between the populations, or a false negative, that is, failure to detect a difference when the level of expression is low owing to poor amplification of the gene. Identification of false positives is less of a concern because of independent methods that are available for confirmation of expression results, such as ISH and RNase protection.

These drawbacks in no way decrease the overall utility of analysis of single-cell expression because the potential gain of knowledge about genes that are significantly differentially expressed between single-cell populations is of vast importance, as evidenced by the significant observations already made by investigators using single cells. Researchers using the technique should be aware of its potential limitations and perform the necessary controls to confirm their results.

## Summary

Recent advances in cDNA array technology have made expression profiling of the brains of patients with neurodegenerative diseases an exciting new approach to understanding the molecular basis of disease. Fluorescent and/or radioisotopic detection of cDNAs or ESTs adhered to a solid support allows for simultaneous assessment of several to hundreds (candidate gene analysis) and thousands (large-scale analysis) of genes. Thus, an unprecedented level of high-throughput genetic analysis is possible for any given neurodegenerative disease. Archived fixed tissue can be an invaluable source of nucleic acids for expression analysis, provided antemortem variables are considered, proper experimental controls are utilized to assess RNA stability, and the limitations of postmortem tissue are recognized.

Further advances toward understanding the mechanism(s) underlying the pathogenesis of neurodegenerative disorders may lie in the ability to combine regional and single-cell expression profiling methodologies with viable and representative in vivo and in vitro models of neuronal degeneration. For example, molecular fingerprints of cell culture manipulations of human-derived neurons and transgenic animals are likely to be the substrates for investigation into mechanisms of selective neuronal degeneration and ultimately are likely to pave the way for novel pharmacotherapeutic interventions and subsequent multicenter clinical trials.

## Acknowledgments

This work was supported by grants from the National Institute on Aging of the National Institutes of Health, and the Alzheimer's Association. We thank Dr. James H. Eberwine, professor of pharmacology and psychiatry at the University of Pennsylvania, for his critical review of this manuscript; Dr. Scott E. Hemby, assistant professor of pharmacology at Emory University; and Dr. Peter Crino, assistant professor of neurology at the University of Pennsylvania. We also wish to acknowledge our colleagues, especially the histotechnologists and neuropathologists, of the Center for Neurodegenerative Disease Research and the Department of Pathology and Laboratory Medicine at the University of Pennsylvania for their assistance and support. We also express our appreciation to the families of the patients studied here who made this research possible. Disclosures: Drs. Lee and Trojanowski are founding scientists of and consult for Layton Biosciences, Inc., the commercial license holder of aRNA amplification and in situ transcription methodologies.

# References

Barton AJ, Pearson RC, and Najlerahim A et al. (1993). Pre- and postmortem influences on brain RNA. *J Neurochem* 61(1): 1–11.

Ben-Ezra J, Johnson DA, and Rossi J et al. (1991). Effect of fixation on the amplification of nucleic acids from paraffin-embedded material by the polymerase chain reaction. *J Histochem Cytochem* 39(3): 351–4.

Bonner RF, Emmert-Buck M, and Cole K et al. (1997). Laser capture microdissection: Molecular analysis of tissue. *Science* 278(5342): 1481, 1483.

Braak H and Braak E (1997). Neuropathological staging of Alzheimer-related changes. *Acta Neuropathol* 82: 239–59.

Brail LH, Jang A, and Billia F et al. (1999). Gene expression in individual cells: Analysis using global single cell reverse transcription polymerase chain reaction (GSC RT-PCR). *Mutat Res* 406(2–4): 45–54.

Brown PO and Botstein D (1999). Exploring the new world of the genome with DNA microarrays. *Nat Genet* 21(Suppl 1): 33–7.

Burton MP, Schneider BG, and Brown R et al. (1998). Comparison of histologic stains for use in PCR analysis of microdissected, paraffin-embedded tissues. *Biotechniques* 24(1): 86–92.

Cheetham JE, Coleman PD, and Chow N (1997). Isolation of single immunohistochemically identified whole neuronal cell bodies from post-mortem human brain for simultaneous analysis of multiple gene expression. *J Neurosci Methods* 77(1): 43–8.

Chiang LW (1998). Detection of gene expression in single neurons by patch-clamp and single-cell reverse transcriptase polymerase chain reaction. *J Chromatogr A* 806(1): 209–18.

Chow N, Cox C, and Callahan LM et al. (1998). Expression profiles of multiple genes in single neurons of Alzheimer's disease. *Proc Natl Acad Sci USA* 95(16): 9620–5.

Colantuoni C, Purcell A, and Christopher MB et al. (2000). High throughput analysis of gene expression in the human brain. *J Neurosci Res* 59: 1–10.

Coombs NJ, Gough AC, and Primrose JN (1999). Optimisation of DNA and RNA extraction from archival formalin-fixed tissue. *Nucleic Acids Res* 27(16): e12.

Crino PB, Trojanowski JQ, and Dichter MA et al. (1996). Embryonic neuronal markers in tuberous sclerosis: Single-cell molecular pathology. *Proc Natl Acad Sci USA* 93(24): 14152–7.

Crino PB, Khodakhah K, and Becker K et al. (1998). Presence and phosphorylation of transcription factors in dendrites. *Proc Natl Acad Sci USA* 95: 2313–18.

Crisan D and Mattson JC (1993). Retrospective DNA analysis using fixed tissue specimens. *DNA Cell Biol* 12(5): 455–64.

Crisan D, Cadoff EM, and Mattson JC et al. (1990). Polymerase chain reaction: Amplification of DNA from fixed tissue. *Clin Biochem* 23(6): 489–95.

Duggan DJ, Bittner M, and Chen Y et al. (1999). Expression profiling using cDNA microarrays. *Nat Genet* 21(Suppl 1): 10–14.

Eberwine J, Spencer C, and Miyashiro K et al. (1992a). Complementary DNA synthesis in situ: Methods and applications. *Methods Enzymol* 216: 80–100.

Eberwine J, Yeh H, and Miyashiro K et al. (1992b). Analysis of gene expression in single live neurons. *Proc Natl Acad Sci USA* 89(7): 3010–14.

Finke J, Fritzen R, and Ternes P et al. (1993). An improved strategy and a useful housekeeping gene for RNA analysis from formalin-fixed, paraffin-embedded tissues by PCR. *Biotechniques* 14(3): 448–53.

Foss RD, Guha-Thakurta N, and Conran RM et al. (1994). Effects of fixative and fixation time on the extraction and polymerase chain reaction amplification of RNA from paraffin-embedded tissue. Comparison of two housekeeping gene mRNA controls. *Diagn Mol Pathol* 3(3): 148–55.

Gall K, Pavelic J, and Jadro-Santel D et al. (1993). DNA amplification by polymerase chain reaction from brain tissues embedded in paraffin. *Int J Exp Pathol* 74(4): 333–7.

Ghasemzadeh MB, Sharma S, and Surmeier DJ et al. (1996). Multiplicity of glutamate receptor subunits in single striatal neurons: An RNA amplification study. *Mol Pharmacol* 49(5): 852–9.

Ginsberg SD, Hemby SE, Lee VM-Y, and Eberwine JH (2000). Expression profile of transcripts in Alzheimer's disease tangle-bearing CA1 neurons. *Ann Neurol* 48(1): 77–87.

Ginsberg SD, Crino PB, and Lee VM et al. (1997). Sequestration of RNA in Alzheimer's disease neurofibrillary tangles and senile plaques. *Ann Neurol* 41(2): 200–9.

Ginsberg SD, Galvin JE, and Chiu T-S et al. (1998). RNA sequestration to pathological lesions of neurodegenerative disorders. *Acta Neuropathol* 96: 487–94.

Ginsberg SD, Crino PB, and Hemby SE et al. (1999a). Predominance of neuronal mRNAs in individual Alzheimer's disease senile plaques. *Ann Neurol* 45(2): 174–81.

Ginsberg SD, Schmidt ML, and Crino PB et al. (1999b). Molecular pathology of Alzheimer's disease and related disorders. In *Cerebral Cortex*, Vol. 14. *Neurodegenerative and Age-related Changes in Structure and Function of Cerebral Cortex*, A. Peters and J. H. Morrison, eds., Kluwer Academic/Plenum, New York, pp. 603–53.

Glowatzki E (1997). Analysis of gene expression in the organ of Corti revealed by single-cell RT-PCR. *Audiol Neurootol* 2(1–2): 71–8.

Glowatzki E, Fakler G, and Brandle U et al. (1995). Subunit-dependent assembly of inward-rectifier K+ channels. *Proc Roy Soc Lond Ser B, Biol Sci* 261(1361): 251–61.

Goldsworthy SM, Stockton PS, and Trempus CS et al. (1999). Effects of fixation on RNA extraction and amplification from laser capture microdissected tissue. *Mol Carcinog* 25(2): 86–91.

Greer CE, Lund JK, and Manos MM (1991a). PCR amplification from paraffin-embedded tissues: Recommendations on fixatives for long-term storage and prospective studies. *PCR Methods Appl* 1(1): 46–50.

Greer CE, Peterson SL, and Kiviat NB et al. (1991b). PCR amplification from paraffin-embedded tissues. Effects of fixative and fixation time. *Am J Clin Pathol* 95(2): 117–24.

Hemby SE, Ginsberg SD, Brunk B, Arnold SE, Trojanowski JQ, and Eberwine JH (2002). Gene expression profile for schizophrenia: Discrete neuron transcription patterns in the entorhinal cortex. *Arch Gen Psychiatry* (in press).

Houts GE, Miyagi M, and Ellis C et al. (1979). Reverse transcriptase from avian myeloblastosis virus. *J Virol* 29(2): 517–22.

Hu M, Krause D, and Greaves M et al. (1997). Multilineage gene expression precedes commitment in the hemopoietic system. *Genes Dev* 11(6): 774–85.

Hyman BT, Van Horsen GW, and Damasio AR et al. (1984). Alzheimer's disease: Cell-specific pathology isolates the hippocampal formation. *Science* 225(4667): 1168–70.

Jackson DP, Quirke P, and Lewis F et al. (1989). Detection of measles virus RNA in paraffin-embedded tissue. *Lancet* 1(8651): 1391.

Jackson DP, Lewis FA, and Taylor GR et al. (1990). Tissue extraction of DNA and RNA and analysis by the polymerase chain reaction. *J Clin Pathol* 43(6): 499–504.

Johnson SA, Morgan DG, and Finch CE (1986). Extensive postmortem stability of RNA from rat and human brain. *J Neurosci Res* 16(1): 267–80.

Johnston NL, Cervenak J, and Shore AD et al. (1997). Multivariate analysis of RNA levels from postmortem human brains as measured by three different methods of RT-PCR. Stanley Neuropathology Consortium. [Published erratum appears in *J Neurosci Meth* Feb 20, 1998; 79(2): 233.] *J Neurosci Meth* 77(1): 83–92.

Kacharmina JE, Crino PB, and Eberwine J (1999). Preparation of cDNA from single cells and subcellular regions. *Methods Enzymol* 303: 3–18.

Kadkol SS, Gage WR, and Pasternack GR (1999). *In situ* hybridization-theory and practice. *Mol Diagn* 4(3): 169–83.

Karsten SL, Van Deerlin VMD, Sabatti C, Gill LH, Geschwind DH (2002). An evaluation of tyramide signal amplification and archived fixed and frozen tissue in microarray gene expression analysis. *Nucleic Acids Res* 30(2): in press.

Kingsbury AE, Foster OJ, and Nisbet AP et al. (1995). Tissue pH as an indicator of mRNA preservation in human post-mortem brain. *Brain Res Mol Brain Res* 28(2): 311–18.

Kontur PJ, Al-Tikriti M, and Innis RB et al. (1994). Postmortem stability of monoamines, their metabolites, and receptor binding in rat brain regions. *J Neurochem* 62: 282–90.

Koopmans M, Monroe SS, and Coffield LM et al. (1993). Optimization of extraction and PCR amplification of RNA extracts from paraffin-embedded tissue in different fixatives. *J Virol Methods* 43(2): 189–204.

Krafft AE, Duncan BW, and Bijwaard KE et al. (1997). Optimization of the isolation and amplification of RNA from formalin-fixed, paraffin-embedded tissue: The Armed Forces Institute of Pathology experience and literature review. *Mol Diagn* 2(3): 217–30.

Leonard S, Logel J, and Luthman D et al. (1993). Biological stability of mRNA isolated from human postmortem brain collections. *Biol Psychiatry* 33(6): 456–66.

Lipshutz RJ, Fodor SP, and Gingeras TR et al. (1999). High density synthetic oligonucleotide arrays. *Nat Genet* 21(Suppl 1): 20–4.

Lockhart DJ, Dong H, and Byrne MC et al. (1996). Expression monitoring by hybridization to high-density oligonucleotide arrays. *Nat Biotechnol* 14(13): 1675–80.

Luo L, Salunga RC, and Guo H et al. (1999). Gene expression profiles of laser-captured adjacent neuronal subtypes. [Published erratum appears in *Nat Med* Mar 1999; 5(3): 355.] *Nat Med* 5(1): 117–22.

Madison RD and Robinson GA (1998). Lambda RNA internal standards quantify sensitivity and amplification efficiency of mammalian gene expression profiling. *Biotechniques* 25(3): 504–8, 510, 512, passim.

Masuda N, Ohnishi T, and Kawamoto S et al. (1999). Analysis of chemical modification of RNA from formalin-fixed samples and optimization of molecular biology applications for such samples. *Nucleic Acids Res* 27(22): 4436–43.

Mizuno T, Nagamura H, and Iwamoto KS et al. (1998). RNA from decades-old archival tissue blocks for retrospective studies. *Diagn Mol Pathol* 7(4): 202–8.

Morrison-Bogorad M, Zimmerman AL, and Pardue S (1995). Heat-shock 70 messenger RNA levels in human brain: Correlation with agonal fever. *J Neurochem* 64(1): 235–46.

Muratori L (1998). *In situ* reverse transcriptase-polymerase chain reaction: An innovative tool for hepatitis C virus RNA detection and localisation, and for quantification of infected cells. *Eur J Histochem* 42(2): 133–6.

Nair SM, Werkman TR, and Craig J et al. (1998). Corticosteroid regulation of ion channel conductances and mRNA levels in individual hippocampal CA1 neurons. *J Neurosci* 18(7): 2685–96.

O'Dell DM, Raghupathi R, and Crino PB et al. (1998). Amplification of mRNAs from single, fixed, TUNEL-positive cells. *Biotechniques* 25(4): 566–8, 570.

Pardue S, Zimmerman AL, and Morrison-Bogorad M (1994). Selective postmortem degradation of inducible heat shock protein 70 (hsp70) mRNAs in rat brain. *Cell Mol Neurobiol* 14(4): 341–57.

Perrett CW, Marchbanks RM, and Whatley SA (1988). Characterisation of messenger RNA extracted post-mortem from the brains of schizophrenic, depressed and control subjects. *J Neurol Neurosurg Psychiatry* 51(3): 325–31.

Phillips J and Eberwine JH (1996). Antisense RNA amplification: A linear amplification method for analyzing the mRNA population from single living cells. *Methods: A Companion to Methods in Enzymology* 10(3): 283–8.

Rappolee DA, Wang A, and Mark D et al. (1989). Novel method for studying mRNA phenotypes in single or small numbers of cells. *J Cell Biochem* 39(1): 1–11.

Ross BM, Knowler JT, and McCulloch J (1992). On the stability of messenger RNA and ribosomal RNA in the brains of control human subjects and patients with Alzheimer's disease. *J Neurochem* 58(5): 1810–19.

Schramm M, Falkai P, and Tepest R et al. (1999). Stability of RNA transcripts in postmortem psychiatric brains. *J Neural Transm* 106(3–4): 329–35.

Shibata D, Kurosu M, and Noguchi TT (1991). Fixed human tissues: A resource for the identification of individuals. *J Forensic Sci* 36(4): 1204–12.

Simone NL, Bonner RF, and Gillespie JW et al. (1998). Laser-capture microdissection: Opening the microscopic frontier to molecular analysis. *Trends Genet* 14(7): 272–6.

Stanta G and Bonin S (1998). RNA quantitative analysis from fixed and paraffin-embedded tissues: Membrane hybridization and capillary electrophoresis. *Biotechniques* 24(2): 271–6.

Stanta G and Schneider C (1991). RNA extracted from paraffin-embedded human tissues is amenable to analysis by PCR amplification. *Biotechniques* 11(3): 304, 306, 308.

Suarez-Quian CA, Goldstein SR, and Pohida T et al. (1999). Laser capture microdissection of single cells from complex tissues. *Biotechniques* 26(2): 328–35.

Tecott LH, Barchas JD, and Eberwine JH (1988). *In situ* transcription: Specific synthesis of complementary DNA in fixed tissue sections. *Science* 240(4859): 1661–4.

Thaker V (1999). *In situ* RT-PCR and hybridization techniques. *Methods Mol Biol* 115: 379–402.

Tong J, Bendahhou S, and Chen H et al. (1994). A simplified method for single-cell RT-PCR that can detect and distinguish genomic DNA and mRNA transcripts. *Nucleic Acids Res* 22(15): 3253–4.

Tournier I, Bernuau D, and Poliard A et al. (1987). Detection of albumin mRNAs in rat liver by *in situ* hybridization: Usefulness of paraffin embedding and comparison of various fixation procedures. *J Histochem Cytochem* 35(4): 453–9.

Van Gelder RN, von Zastrow ME, and Yool A et al. (1990). Amplified RNA synthesized from limited quantities of heterogeneous cDNA. *Proc Natl Acad Sci USA* 87(5): 1663–7.

von Weizsacker F, Labeit S, and Koch HK et al. (1991). A simple and rapid method for the detection of RNA in formalin-fixed, paraffin-embedded tissues by PCR amplification. *Biochem Biophys Res Commun* 174(1): 176–80.

Weiss LM and Chen YY (1991). Effects of different fixatives on detection of nucleic acids from paraffin-embedded tissues by *in situ* hybridization using oligonucleotide probes. *J Histochem Cytochem* 39(9): 1237–42.

West MJ, Coleman PD, and Flood DG et al. (1994). Differences in the pattern of hippocampal neuronal loss in normal ageing and Alzheimer's disease. *Lancet* 344(8925): 769–72.

Zhou CJ, Kikuyama S, and Shibanuma M et al. (2000). Cellular distribution of the splice variants of the receptor for pituitary adenylate cyclase-activating polypeptide [PAC(1)-R] in the rat brain by *in situ* RT-PCR. *Brain Res Mol Brain Res* 75(1): 150–8.

Zhuang Z, Bertheau P, and Emmert-Buck MR et al. (1995). A microdissection technique for archival DNA analysis of specific cell populations in lesions < 1 mm in size. *Am J Pathol* 146(3): 620–5.

# 9 Development of Microarrays to Study Gene Expression in Tissue and Single Cells: Analysis of Neural Transmission

*Marie-Claude Potier, Nathalie Gibelin, Bruno Cauli, Béatrice Le Bourdellès, Bertrand Lambolez, Geoffroy Golfier, Sonia Kuhlmann, Philippe Marc, Fréderic Devaux, and Jean Rossier*

DNA microarrays are used to measure the expression patterns of thousands of genes in parallel, providing a sensitive, global read-out of the physiological state of a cell or tissue sample and generating clues to gene functions. They are also used to monitor changes in gene expression in response to any physiological, pathological, or pharmacological variations.

With the very high degree of complexity of the brain, this new technology applied at the single-cell level should help in classifying cells according to their gene contents and define new targets for therapeutic intervention. By correlating gene expression with specific physiological properties, it is possible to gain mechanistic insight into a broad range of neurobiological processes. With the single-cell reverse transcription-multiplex PCR (RT-MPCR) technique developed in our laboratory, it is now possible to follow the expression of 20 to 30 genes in individual neurons (Lambolez et al., 1992, 1996; Angulo et al., 1997; Cauli et al., 1997; Porter et al., 1998, 1999). We have been able to correlate electrophysiological properties of interneurons with the expression of neurotransmitters. For example, neocortical interneurons showing an irregular spiking express vasoactive intestinal peptide (VIP), a regulator of metabolism and cerebral blood flow.

We are using the DNA microarray technology on microscope slides developed by Patrick Brown at Stanford University (Schena et al., 1995; Eisen and Brown, 1999). In this technology, DNA molecules are spotted on poly-L-lysine-coated slides. Two spotting machines are routinely used—one from GeneMachines (California) with MicroQuill 1000 from Majer Precision, Inc. making spots by contact with glass; and one from Gesim (Germany) with a piezo-electric device included inside a picoliter pipette.

After hybridization of the microarrays with fluorescent probes (PCR products, cDNAs), the slides are analyzed on a scanner (Scan-Array 3000) from Packard Biosciences that is capable of analyzing Cy3 and Cy5 fluorescence on spots at a resolution of 10 μm per pixel. The scanner is connected to a computer with image analysis software: ImaGene 3 (BioDiscovery Inc.) and Scanalyze 2.32 (M. Eisen, cgm.stanford.edu/pbrown). Steady-state mRNA levels are deduced from the fluorescence intensity at each position on the microarray. With this technology and these machines, it is possible to produce DNA microarrays of low or high density (hundreds, thousands or ten of thousands of spots) on up to 100 slides in the same spotting experiment.

### Description of the DNA Microarrays: A Focused Neurochip

We have developed DNA chips containing 94 PCR fragments of 200 to 600 bp, corresponding to 94 rat genes important in neuro-transmission. These Neurochips include precursors for neuropeptides, enzymes involved in the synthesis of neurotransmitters, calcium-binding proteins, and subunits of receptors for neurotransmitters: glutamate, $\gamma$-aminobutyric acid (GABA), acetylcholine, serotonin, dopamine, and adrenalin (table 9.1). PCR fragments usually correspond to open reading frames (several exons when possible) and are able to differentiate between most of the members within a gene family. These rat Neurochips have been shown to work with human and mouse mRNA samples. The list of gene fragments and PCR primers ($T_m$ between 55 and 65 °C) can be obtained from the web site www.espci.biologie.fr.

PCR fragments (DNA targets) of each of the 94 rat genes were first amplified from 15-day-old rat brain cDNAs and then reamplified and purified on Qiaquick columns (Qiagen). The final concentration of DNA targets before spotting was 100 ng/μl in 3× SSC. All

**Table 9.1**  Genes contained on the Neurochips

| | |
|---|---|
| Calcium binding proteins (3) | Calbindin, parvalbumin, calretinin |
| Enzymes synthesis (8) | GAD65, GAD67, CAT, TH, TpH, NOS-1, NOS-2, NOS-3 |
| Peptides (6) | NPY, VIP, somatostatine, CCK, endorphin, enkephalin |
| AMPA receptors (4) | GluR1, GluR2, GluR3, GluR4 |
| Kainate receptors (5) | KA1, KA2, GluR5, GluR6, GluR7 |
| NMDA receptors (4)[a] | NR2A, NR2B, NR2C, NR2D |
| Metabotropic receptors (8) | mGluR1, mGluR2, mGluR3, mGluR4, mGluR5, mGluR6, mGluR7, mGluR8 |
| GABA receptors (13) | $\alpha1, \alpha2, \alpha3, \alpha4, \alpha5, \alpha6, \beta1, \beta2, \beta3, \gamma1, \gamma2, \gamma3, \delta1$ |
| Nicotinic receptors (10) | $\alpha2, \alpha3, \alpha4, \alpha5, \alpha6, \alpha7, \alpha9, \beta2, \beta3, \beta4$ |
| Muscarinic receptors (5) | m1, m2, m3, m4, m5 |
| Dopamine receptors (5) | D1, D2, D3, D4, D5 |
| 5-HT receptors (13)[b] | 5-HT1A, 5-HT1B, 5-HT1D, 5-HT1E/F, 5-HT2A, 5-HT2B, 5-HT2C, 5-HT3, 5-HT4, 5-HT5a, 5-HT5b, 5-HT6, 5-HT7 |
| Adrenaline receptors (9) | $\alpha1a, \alpha1b, \alpha1c, \alpha2b, \alpha2c, \alpha2d, \beta1, \beta2, \beta3$ |
| Controls (1) | Somatostatine intron |
| Normalizing genes (5) | G3PDH, tubulin, actin, ubiquitin, HPRT |

[a] *N*-methyl-D-aspartate.
[b] 5-hydroxytryptamine.

the DNA targets were reamplified similarly, indicating that the 94 PCR reactions worked efficiently.

For genes within a multigene family, the percentage of identity was calculated. Table 9.2 gives the results for the AMPA-kainate family. The asymmetry of the table is due to the variable positions of DNA targets along the 3′- to 5′-axis of genes. We have hybridized a 2540-bp fluorescent PCR probe corresponding to the GluR3 subunit to microarrays containing all the AMPA and kainate receptor subunits listed in table 9.2 at various stringency conditions (e.g., hybridization buffer and temperature, washing buffer and temperature).

**Table 9.2** Percentage of homology between DNA targets (horizontal column) and the corresponding DNA fragments in the genes of the same family (vertical column)

|       | GluR1 | GluR2 | GluR3 | GluR4 | GluR5 | GluR6 | GluR7 | Ka1 | Ka2 |
|-------|-------|-------|-------|-------|-------|-------|-------|-----|-----|
| GluR1 |       | 54%   | 53%   | 53%   | 45%   | 42%   | 41%   | 38% | 38% |
| GluR2 | 60%   |       | 60%   | 62%   | 39%   | 37%   | 37%   | 34% | 33% |
| GluR3 | 73%   | 74%   |       | 75%   | 56%   | 61%   | 55%   | 55% | 53% |
| GluR4 | 77%   | 76%   | 81%   |       | 45%   | 47%   | 46%   | 45% | 46% |
| GluR5 | 61%   | 60%   | 60%   | 60%   |       | 81%   | 80%   | 65% | 67% |
| GluR6 | 36%   | 38%   | 39%   | 41%   | 65%   |       | 53%   | 41% | 40% |
| GluR7 | 39%   | 40%   | 39%   | 36%   | 70%   | 72%   |       | 40% | 41% |
| Ka1   | 36%   | 34%   | 35%   | 35%   | 37%   | 38%   | 37%   |     | 61% |
| Ka2   | 36%   | 36%   | 37%   | 34%   | 41%   | 40%   | 43%   | 69% |     |

Cross-hybridizations do occur with GluR2 and GluR4 subunits, but such cross-hybridizations are at the lowest when (1) an SSC/SDS buffer (3.5× SSC, 0.3% SDS) at 60 °C is used instead of a 50% formamide buffer at 42 °C, and (2) when the slides are washed at 65 °C in 0.05× SSC. No cross-hybridization was detected with GluR1 despite 73% homology with GluR3. The difference in cross-hybridization observed between GluR1 and GluR2-GluR4 can be explained by the location of homology within the DNA sequence. A 70% homology can correspond to either a 70% homology evenly distributed along the DNA sequence or to a 100% homology in 70% of the sequence. For minimizing cross-hybridization within multigene families, the percentage of identity should be less than 70% and as homogeneously distributed as possible.

## Analysis of Gene Expression in Whole Brain Tissue with the Neurochip

Differential expression using cDNAs from tissue samples labeled with a fluorochrome (Cy5) during reverse transcription of mRNAs hybridized to the arrays together with cDNAs from a control tissue labeled with another fluorochrome (Cy3) can be measured with the Neurochips. It is possible to detect a 1.5-fold variation in the level of expression of any gene that is sufficiently transcribed. A standard amount of cDNA (equivalent to 1 μg of polyA$^+$ mRNA) is necessary to get a strong fluorescent signal without use of signal amplification techniques. For cDNA labeling and microarray hybridization, we followed the protocols from the Brown laboratory (available at cgm.stanford.edu/pbrown).

In collaboration with the Neuroscience Research Center of Merck Sharp & Dohme (B. Le Bourdellès, T. Rosahl, and P. Whiting), we have studied the expression pattern of the 94 genes contained on the Neurochip in mice in which the $\beta$2 subunit of the GABA-A receptor was knocked out (KO). The most prominent GABA-A receptor combination in mammalian brain is $\alpha 1/\beta 2/\gamma 2$. In the $\beta$2 KO adult mice, about 50% of $^3$H-Flumazenil binding sites are lost. However the $\beta$2 homozygotes appear phenotypically normal, with a slightly increased activity. A 50% loss of inhibitory receptors could be compensated for by an under- or overexpression of other receptors, resulting in the absence of a severe phenotype in the animals. We used the Neurochip for studying a putative compensatory mechanism (figure 9.1 and plate 6). Experiments were performed on two adult animals (at least 7 months old). For the normalization of the experiments we added actin, tubulin, hypoxanthine-guanine phosphoribosyl transferase (HPRT), ubiquitin, and reduced glucose-3-phosphate dehydrogenase (G3PDH) DNA targets onto the Neurochips. The G3PDH was found to be the best normalizing gene in rat brain, despite its high level of expression compared with most of the genes present on the Neurochip.

The $\beta$2 subunit is still transcribed in the KO mice because of the construct design. A neomycin cassette was introduced in the $\beta$2 subunit gene that did not completely suppress the transcription, but resulted in an inhibition of translation of mRNAs into proteins. In addition, we have detected a reproducible downregulation of

A

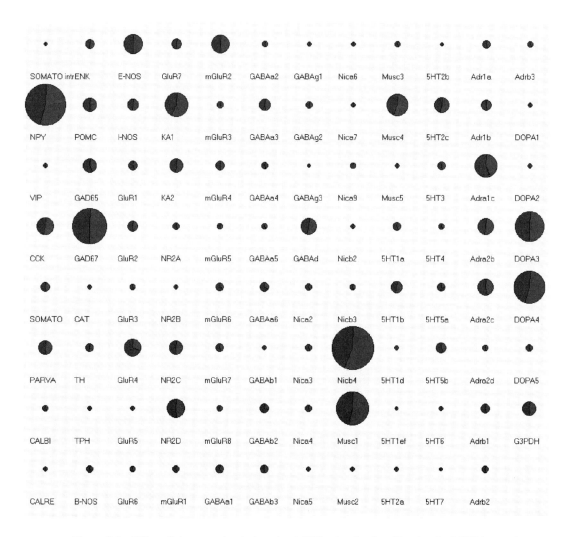

**Figure 9.1** Differential expression in knockout (KO) mice for the $\beta$2-subunit of GABA receptors of the 94 genes present on the Neurochips (*A*) or a subset of GABA-A receptor subunits (*B*). (*A*) An example of the results obtained: the pies correspond to the differential expression in KO mice (red) vs. control mice (green). (*B*) A selection of all the

B

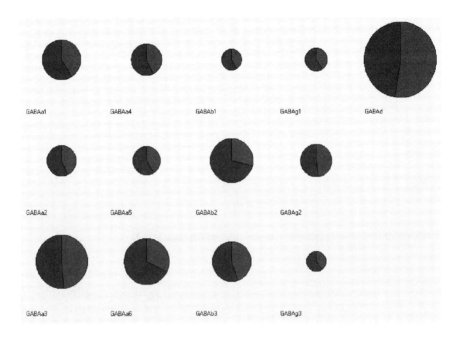

GABA-A receptor subunits. Pies were calculated using a program written by P. Marc and C. Jacq from the Ecole Normale Superieure in Paris (www.biologie.ens.fr/ microarrays.html). The size of the pies is proportional to the sum of fluorescence intensities in KO and control mice. In (*B*) it can be seen that the $\beta$2 subunit is downregulated together with other subunits, among which some are clustered on the same chromosome in the order $\beta$2 $\alpha$6-$\alpha$1 $\gamma$2 in humans (Kostrzewa et al., 1996). See plate 6 for color version.

the calcium-binding proteins calbindin and calretinin with a ratio greater than 1.5. The glutamate receptor subunits GluR4, GluR6, and mGluR6; muscarinic receptor 2; and the 5-HT5a (5-hydroxy-L-tryptophan) serotonin receptor could also be downregulated. We have compared the ratios obtained for GABA-A receptor subunits $\alpha$1, $\alpha$6, and $\gamma$2 using Neurochips and Northern blots (table 9.3). The expression ratios on Northern blots confirmed the Neurochip data.

**Table 9.3** Comparison of the ratios of expression of various GABA-A receptor subunits using Neurochips or Northern blots in control versus β2-KO mice

| GABA-A RECEPTOR SUBUNIT | NEUROCHIPS | NORTHERN BLOTS |
|---|---|---|
| α1 | 0.69–0.66 | 0.65 |
| α6 | 0.47–0.5 | 0.22–0.21 |
| β2 | 0.39–0.21 | ND[a] |
| γ2 | 0.91–0.71 | 1.13 |

[a] ND, Nondetermined.

### Analysis of Gene Expression in Single Cells using Neurochips

The single-cell RT-PCR method was developed in our laboratory in 1992 by B. Lambolez and E. Audinat (Lambolez et al., 1992). This technique allows the correlation of electrophysiological properties of single neurons with gene expression within that cell. Using RT-multiplex-PCR, it is possible to analyze 30 genes in a single cell (Cauli et al., 1997). After patch clamp recording, the cytoplasm of the cell is harvested through the recording pipette and the mRNA content is reverse transcribed into cDNAs. The cDNAs are amplified in two rounds of PCR. The first round is a 20-cycle multiplex PCR that simultaneously amplifies all of the 30 genes. The second round consists of 30 different PCRs, each one specific for one of the 30 genes. The PCR products of the second round have to be analyzed by agarose gel electrophoresis (figure 9.2).

For studying a larger number of genes at the single-cell level, we are now using the Neurochip. In order to test the multiplex PCR for amplifying 94 genes in the same reaction, we performed some hybridization with mRNAs or cDNAs from the same 15-day-old rat brain. Experiments were done at least twice on two different sets of microarrays obtained from different batches of DNA targets spotted with the two spotters described earlier.

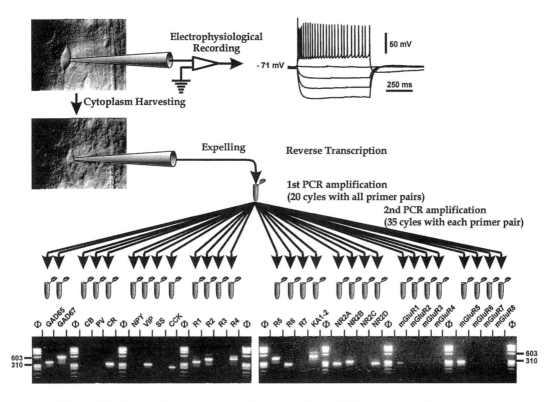

**Figure 9.2** Protocol for reverse transcriptase-/multiplex PCR from single cells.

The 94 DNA targets were amplified in 94 separate PCR reactions from cDNA quantities corresponding to a one-cell content (the equivalent of about 1 pg of mRNA). The PCR products were analyzed on agarose gels. A band that was not detectable was given a value of 1. Values 2, 3, 4, and 5 were assigned to genes giving, respectively, low, medium, high, and very high intensity bands on agarose gel after staining with ethidium bromide. This experiment is called ''agarose RT-PCR'' (see figures 9.3 and 9.4, axis 2; see also plate 6).

In another experiment, the 94 DNA targets were amplified in 94 separate PCR reactions in which Cy5-dCTP was incorporated. Fluorescent DNA targets were mixed, purified on a Qiaquick column,

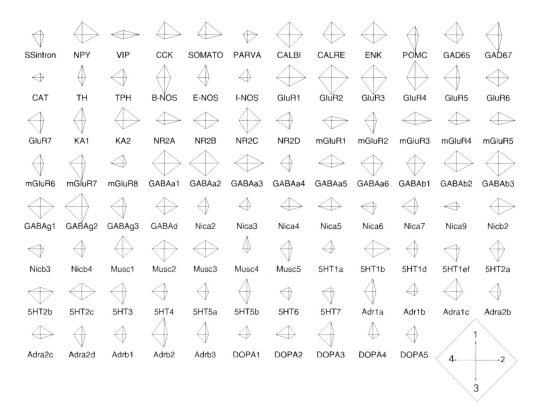

**Figure 9.3** Star plot for analyzing hybridization to the Neurochip. Axis 1, fluorescent cDNAs; axis 2, agarose RT-PCR; axis 3, size of the DNA targets; axis 4, fluorescent PCR probe.

and hybridized to the Neurochip in $3.5\times$ SSC/0.3% SDS at $60\,^{\circ}$C in a humid chamber overnight. The Neurochip was then washed at room temperature in $0.05\times$ SSC, and the fluorescent signal was analyzed on the ScanArray 3000 (Packard Biosciences). A fluorescent signal of up to 3000 per spot was given the value 1; from 3000 to 10,000, the value 2; from 10,000 to 30,000, the value 3; from 30,000 to 50,000, the value 4; and from 50,000 to 65,534, the value 5. This experiment is called the "fluorescent PCR probe" (see figure 9.3, axis 4).

We then amplified the 94 genes in a multiplex PCR in one tube. A total of 10 fg of each DNA target were mixed and amplified in one 100-μl, 45-cycle multiplex PCR experiment (containing the 94 primer pairs [10 pmoles each], 3.5 mM MgCl$_2$, 200 μM dATP and dGTP, 160 μM dTTP and dCTP, and 40 μM Cy3-dCTP and Cy3-dUTP). We used Advantaq from Clontech in the Qiagen Taq buffer containing KCl and (NH$_4$)$_2$SO$_4$, which provides a wider temperature window for specific annealing of primers and a greater tolerance to variable Mg$^{2+}$ concentration. Fluorescent PCR fragments were purified on a Qiaquick column (Qiagen) and eluted in 30 μl of TE. Ten microliters were adjusted to 3.5× SSC and 0.3% SDS (final concentrations) and hybridized to the Neurochip and analyzed as described earlier. This experiment is named "multiplex PCR from DNA targets" (see figure 9.4, axis 1).

The same multiplex PCR was performed starting from cDNA quantities corresponding to a one-cell content (the equivalent of about 1 pg of mRNA). This experiment is named "multiplex PCR from cDNA" (see figure 9.4, axis 3).

In addition, fluorescent cDNAs produced from the same mRNA batch were hybridized to the Neurochip as described earlier. This last experiment is named "fluorescent cDNAs" (see figure 9.3, axis 1).

All these experiments were analyzed using the R software available under the GNU General Public License at gnu.org. In figure 9.3, the size of the DNA target was added (1 for 0 to 200 bp, 2 for 200 to 300 bp, 3 for 300 to 400 bp, 4 for 400 to 500 bp and 5 for 500 to 600 bp) (see figure 9.3, axis 1).

Figure 9.3 shows that the hybridization signal of a mixture of fluorescent target DNAs ("fluorescent PCR probe") is not correlated to the length of the target DNA. For example, a DNA target corresponding to the VIP gene, 287 bp long, gives a high fluorescent hybridization signal, whereas a DNA target corresponding to parvalbumin (PARVA), 388 bp long, gives a low signal. From this first series of experiments, we can identify DNA targets that perform

A

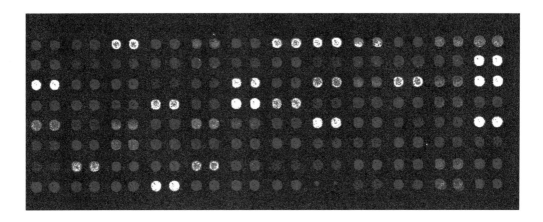

B

| | | | | | | | | | | | |
|---|---|---|---|---|---|---|---|---|---|---|---|
| SSintron | NPY | VIP | CCK | SOMATO | PARVA | CALBI | CALRE | ENK | POMC | GAD65 | GAD67 |
| CAT | TH | TPH | B-NOS | E-NOS | I-NOS | GluR1 | GluR2 | GluR3 | GluR4 | GluR5 | GluR6 |
| GluR7 | KA1 | KA2 | NR2A | NR2B | NR2C | NR2D | mGluR1 | mGluR2 | mGluR3 | mGluR4 | mGluR5 |
| mGluR6 | mGluR7 | mGluR8 | GABAa1 | GABAa2 | GABAa3 | GABAa4 | GABAa5 | GABAa6 | GABAb1 | GABAb2 | GABAb3 |
| GABAg1 | GABAg2 | GABAg3 | GABAd | Nica2 | Nica3 | Nica4 | Nica5 | Nica6 | Nica7 | Nica9 | Nicb2 |
| Nicb3 | Nicb4 | Musc1 | Musc2 | Musc3 | Musc4 | Musc5 | 5HT1a | 5HT1b | 5HT1d | 5HT1ef | 5HT2a |
| 5HT2b | 5HT2c | 5HT3 | 5HT4 | 5HT5a | 5HT5b | 5HT6 | 5HT7 | Adr1a | Adr1b | Adra1c | Adra2b |
| Adra2c | Adra2d | Adrb1 | Adrb2 | Adrb3 | DOPA1 | DOPA2 | DOPA3 | DOPA4 | DOPA5 | | |

poorly and then choose another primer set for gene amplification in the corresponding gene sequence. This process can be repeated until the signal is optimized.

Figure 9.4A shows an example of Neurochip hybridization of the fluorescent multiplex PCR products obtained from cDNA quantities corresponding to a one-cell content. The microtiter platelike organization of the genes in figure 9.3 and figure 9.4B corresponds to the order of spotting in figure 9.4A, where genes were spotted in duplicates.

Twenty genes (underlined) out of 94 were not correctly amplified in the "multiplex PCR from DNA targets" experiment (figure 9.4). When expressed in rat brain and detected in the "agarose RT-PCR" experiment, these 20 genes will not be detected in the multiplex experiments. Figure 9.4B also shows that some genes give perfect equilateral triangles. Although a multiplex PCR for amplifying 94 genes in the same reaction will never be quantitative, we observed that the expression levels of 12 genes are largely underestimated. One example is GluR1, for which the hybridization of fluorescent cDNAs or a fluorescent PCR probe is correct (figure 9.3), but the multiplex PCR is not very efficient (figure 9.4).

Finally, for three genes—GluR7, GAD67, and Adr$\beta$2—the expression levels deduced from hybridization of fluorescent cDNAs are higher than those from agarose RT-PCR experiments (figure 9.3). For GAD67, the discrepancy could be explained by a cross-hybridization with GAD65, for GluR7 by a cross-hybridization with GluR5 (although the expression of GluR5 is not very high), and for Adr$\beta$2 by a cross-hybridization with another gene.

**Figure 9.4** (*A*) Hybridization to the Neurochip of multiplex PCR products obtained from cDNA quantities corresponding to a one-cell content. The spectrum of colors corresponds to the level of fluorescent signal: from black-blue to white for increasing intensities. (*B*) Star plot for analyzing multiplex PCR for amplifying 94 genes in one tube. Axis 1, multiplex PCR from DNA targets; axis 2, agarose RT-PCR; axis 3, multiplex PCR from cDNA corresponding to (*A*). See plate 7 for color version.

## Conclusions

In a fashion similar to the development of PCR or recombinant DNA technology, microarrays have a large number of applications that will expand over time. In neurobiology, because of the great cellular diversity of the brain, it is important to develop techniques that will be applied to the study of gene expression at the single-cell level. Since the mRNA content of individual cells is much less complex than the mRNA content of a whole brain, it can be predicted that the multiplex PCR protocol can be used for amplifying 74 genes from individual cells in one reaction and hybridizing fluorescent PCR products to the Neurochip. These experiments will provide yes or no answers, but not quantitative data. An alternative is the protocol described in figure 9.2 for amplifying 94 genes from a single cell in two steps: the first step by multiplex PCR in one tube and the second step by 94 individual PCRs in a microtiter plate. This protocol has been used for analyzing the expression profile of Purkinje cells.

It is important when designing new microarrays to work out the problem of specificity between members of large gene families. This has been ignored in most large microarray designs. With RT-PCR, specificity relies on the sequence of the primer pairs. With DNA microarrays, specificity relies on the sequence of the hundreds of DNA targets.

## Acknowledgments

The authors would like to thank Mike Eisen for very useful advice and Alex Papanastassiou for participating in the production of DNA targets. This work was supported by Centre National de la Recherche Scientifique (Genome Project), Association de Recherche sur le Cancer, and Curie Institute Funds.

**Protocol:** Materials and methods for single-cell RT-PCR

### Solutions

- Diluting buffer: Tris HCl,10 mM, pH 8 autoclaved solution
- Patch intracellular solution: 140 mM CsCl, 3 mM $MgCl_2$, 5 mM EGTA, 10 mM HEPES (pH 7.2). Eighty milligrams of this solution are prepared as follows: CsCl, $MgCl_2$, and HEPES are dissolved in 60 ml of water and 2 ml of the EGTA (200 mM dissolved in 0.1 N KOH) stock solution are added. The pH is adjusted to 7.2 with KOH. The volume is then adjusted to 80 ml with water and the solution is filtered (to remove any particle that may preclude gigaohm sealing) and autoclaved; 1-ml aliquots are then stored at $-80\,°C$ until use. It is possible to replace CsCl with 140 mM KCl or potassium gluconate. In addition, neuronal tracers such as biocytin may be added in the patch intracellular solution to achieve morphological analysis. The composition of this intracellular solution may be changed. For instance, the $MgCl_2$ concentration can be decreased and $MgCl_2$ can be added afterward to the RT reaction if necessary, to reach a final concentration of 2 mM. In theory, any patch pipette solution can be used, provided it does not contain inhibitors of the RT or PCR reaction. Since the RT reaction takes place after the recording, the final concentration of the reagents can be adjusted accordingly.
- $20\times$ DTT (Dithiothreitol): A 1 M solution is prepared in water and filtered (millex). The working solution ($20\times$) is 0.2 M in water stored as 50-μl aliquots in 1.5-ml screw-cap tubes under nitrogen at $-80\,°C$.
- $5\times$ RT mix: Hexamer random primers (Boehringer Mannheim) are dissolved in Tris, 10 mM, pH 8, at 5 mM. Deoxyribonucleotides (dNTPs) (Pharmacia) are each supplied as a 100 mM solution. A working RT mix solution ($5\times$) of random primers and dNTPs is prepared in Tris, 10 mM, pH 8, with random primers at 25 μM and dNTPs at 2.5 mM each. This working mix is stored as 30-μl aliquots in 500-μl tubes at $-20\,°C$.
- RNAsin and reverse transcriptase (RTase, SSII from Gibco BRL) are both stored at $-80\,°C$, each as 5-μl aliquots in 1.5-ml screw-cap tubes under nitrogen.
- PCR buffers: The $10\times$ Taq buffer supplied by Perkin Elmer or Qiagen with 15 mM $MgCl_2$ included was found suitable for all our PCR reactions.
- $100\times$ dNTP PCR solution: This solution contains the four dNTPs, each at 5 mM, in 10 mM Tris pH 8. This solution is used for the reamplification of the products from the first PCR or in pilot experiments.
- $100\times$ PCR oligonucleotide primer: The stock is kept at $-20\,°C$, undiluted. The working solution ($100\times$) is diluted at 10 pmol/μl (for $100\times$) in Tris, 10 mM, pH 8. This $100\times$ solution is stored in 50-μl aliquots at $-20\,°C$.

- 200× PCR oligonucleotide primer and multiplex primer premix: When multiplexing involves a large number of primer pairs (for instance, 10 pairs), we prepare a 200× working solution for each separate primer as described above (20 pmol/μl) and mix equal volumes of each primer to prepare a premix: for 10 primer pairs (20 primers), we use 10 μl of this premix for each reaction tube (10 pmol of each primer).
- PCR primer design: The choice of the oligos is especially important. In most instances, failure in pilot experiments can be related to poor design of a primer pair (with stable hairpin or primer-dimer). For multiplex PCR, the melting point of all primers must be between 55 and 60 °C. We selected primers generating cDNA-amplified fragments ranging from about 200 to 600 bp. In order to avoid genomic DNA amplification from the nucleus, oligonucleotide primers are designed on separate exons. If the gene structure is not known, we proceed to amplifications of 200 ng genomic DNA and compare it with the cDNA amplification product.

### Harvesting procedure

The very first step of the single-cell RT-PCR protocol starts with the electrophysiological recording of the neuron to be analyzed. The cell is first visually identified and chosen according to morphological criteria. The patch pipette filled with 8 μl of intracellular solution is then moved toward the neuron with a positive pressure to avoid contamination by the surrounding tissue.

Once the pipette reaches the neuron, a gigaohm seal is made, which ensures a very tight contact between the cell membrane and the pipette, avoiding the risk of contamination (cell-attached configuration). The patch membrane under the pipette is then broken by applying a brief negative pressure, establishing a physical and electrical continuity between the cytoplasm and the pipette solution. At the end of the recording, the cell's content is aspirated into the recording pipette under electrophysiological and visual control to avoid contamination and to ensure a good cytoplasm collection. The harvesting procedure is stopped if the gigaohm seal is lost. After the cytoplasm is collected, the pipette is gently withdrawn from the neuron to favor the closure of the cell membrane. Ideally, an outside-out configuration is then achieved, which allows the preservation of the pipette's content.

The electrophysiological control of this harvesting procedure offers several advantages over laser capture microdissection, another single-cell collecting technique. First, only the mRNAs from the recorded neuron are harvested, with very limited risk of contamination by the tissue surrounding the cell. Second, the harvesting procedure allows a good preservation of the collected mRNAs. Third and inherent to the single-cell RT-PCR technique, the analyzed neuron can be electrophysiologically and pharmacologically characterized. Finally, when a diffusible tracer (e.g., biocytin) is added to the patch solution, a detailed morphology of the neuron can be obtained for further anatomical identification.

### General protocol for the RT reaction

During the course of the electrophysiological experiments, the aliquots of intracellular solution, $5\times$ RT mix, and $20\times$ DTT are kept on ice, and RNAsin and RTase are kept at $-20\,°C$. During the recording, 2 µl of $5\times$ RT mix and 0.5 µl of $20\times$ DTT are pipetted into the RT-PCR tube. After the cell is recorded and aspirated, the pipette's content is expelled (we usually expel 6.5 µl) in this tube. We then add 0.5 µl RNAsin and 0.5 µl RTase and the tube is flicked and briefly centrifuged. The final volume should then be roughly 10 µl, with final concentrations of: 0.5 mM each dNTP, 5 µM random primers, 10 mM DTT; and 20 units of RNAsin and 100 units of RTase. The capped tube is then stored overnight at $37\,°C$. After this incubation, the tube is kept at $-80\,°C$ until the PCR reaction.

### General protocol for the first PCR

Hot start always gives better results and is routinely used in our lab. Primers are added in the preheated RT-PCR tubes since primer-dimers are mainly due to the RTase present in the 10-µl RT reaction. We prepare two different solutions. The volume of solution 1 is 70 µl $\times$ number of cell tubes. It contains per cell tube: 10 µl $10\times$ PCR buffer, 0.5 µl Taq polymerase (2.5 units) and water to 70 µl. The volume of solution 2 is 20 µl $\times$ number of cell tubes. It contains per cell tube: 1 µl of the $100\times$ sense primer solution, 1 µl of the $100\times$ antisense primer solution (in case of multiplex, 10 pmol of each primer) and water to 20 µl. Seventy microliters of solution 1 are added to the 10-µl RT reaction in each cell tube and overlaid with 2 drops of mineral oil. The tubes are then placed in the PCR machine preheated to $94\,°C$, and after 1 minute 20 µl of solution 2 are added to each tube on top of the oil. After 1 minute, the PCR program is started.

The final aqueous volume is 100 µl, with the following final concentrations: 50 µM for each dNTP (from the RT reaction), 10 pmol/100 µl of each of the primers, 2.5 units/100 µl of Taq polymerase.

For PCR with only one primer pair, we perform 40 PCR cycles; the amplification products are analyzed by gel electrophoresis with ethidium bromide staining. For multiplex PCR, 20 PCR cycles are performed, followed by a 35-cycle PCR with only one primer pair.

### General protocol for the second PCR

For multiplex PCR (up to 40 primer pairs), we used 0.5–2 µl of the first PCR reaction, without any purification, as template for the second PCR. Each of the cDNA species coamplified during the first PCR is amplified independently by the second PCR. To the 2 µl of the first PCR reaction, 78 ml are added containing per tube, 10 µl $10\times$ Taq buffer, 0.5 µl Taq, 1 µl of the $100\times$ dNTP solution and water. Two drops of oil are added. The tubes are then placed in the PCR machine preheated to $94\,°C$ (hot start protocol), and after 1 minute 20 µl containing 1 µl of the $100\times$ antisense primer solution and water are added to each tube on top of the oil. After 1 minute the PCR program is started. Thirty-five cycles are performed. The products of these second PCR amplifications are then analyzed by agarose gel electrophoresis stained with ethidium bromide.

# References

Angulo MC, Lambolez B, Audinat E, Hestrin S, and Rossier J (1997). Subunit composition, kinetic, and permeation properties of AMPA receptors in single neocortical nonpyramidal cells. *J Neurosci* 17: 6685–96.

Cauli B, Audinat E, Lambolez B, Angulo MC, Ropert N, Tsuzuki K, Hestrin S, and Rossier J (1997). Molecular and physiological diversity of cortical nonpyramidal cells. *J Neurosci* 17: 3894–3906.

Eisen M and Brown P (1999). DNA arrays for analysis of gene expression. *Methods Enzymol* 303: 179–205.

Kostrzewa M, Köhler A, Eppelt K, Hellam L, Fairweather ND, Levy ER, Monaco AP, and Müller U (1996). Assignment of genes encoding GABA-A receptors subunits α1, α6, β2 and γ2 to a YAC contig of 5q33. *Eur J Hum Genet* 4: 199–204.

Lambolez B, Audinat E, Bochet P, Crépel F, and Rossier J (1992). AMPA receptor subunits expressed by single Purkinje cells. *Neuron* 9: 247–58.

Lambolez B, Ropert N, Perrais D, Rossier J, and Hestrin S (1996). Correlation between kinetics and RNA splicing of alpha-amino-3-hydroxy-5-methylisoxazole-4-propionic acid receptors in neocortical neurons. *Proc Nat Acad Sci USA* 93: 1797–1802.

Porter JT, Cauli B, Staiger JF, Lambolez B, Rossier J, and Audinat E (1998). Properties of bipolar VIPergic interneurons and their excitation by pyramidal neurons in the rat neocortex. *Eur J Neurosci* 10: 3617–28.

Porter JT, Cauli B, Tsuzuki K, Lambolez B, Rossier J, and Audinat E (1999). Selective excitation of subtypes of neocortical interneurons by nicotinic receptors. *J Neurosci* 19: 5228–35.

Schena M, Shalon D, Davis R, and Brown P (1995). Quantitative monitoring of gene expression patterns with a complementary DNA microarray. *Science* 270: 467–70.

# 10 Custom cDNA Microarrays Derived from Subtracted Libraries for Neural Gene Discovery and Expression Analysis

*Daniel H. Geschwind and Stanley F. Nelson*

Methods for the analysis of differential gene expression in the nervous system can be artificially divided into techniques that exploit the analysis of known genes and those that focus on gene discovery. The focus of this chapter is the use of DNA microarrays as a screening tool to identify novel genes. Microarrays have been added as a gene screening tool to improve the efficiency and power of cDNA subtractions (Welford et al., 1998; Nelson and Denny, 1999; Yang et al., 1999). The use of cDNA subtraction methods in tandem with DNA microarrays allows efficient comparisons of heterogeneous tissues or cell types of the complexity found in the developing or mature nervous system. These techniques clearly have the power to identify differentially expressed genes of the rarest class, which are expressed in only a subset of cells in a given tissue.

The standard microarray experiment depends upon gridding down known cDNAs or ESTs representing known genes (Schena et al., 1995; DeRisi et al., 1996; Shalon et al., 1996), or genomic clones (DeRisi et al., 1996; Geschwind et al., 1998a). This limits the analysis of gene expression to known genes, which currently account for an estimated 50–60% of genes expressed in the nervous system. The largest collection of commercially available expressed sequence tags is about 40,000. Although eventually all genes will be included on microarrays, such coverage is not currently available. While this represents the state of the art, about half of all genes, especially those of low abundance, remain unidentified. Since these low-abundance genes are most likely to be those contributing to important aspects of neuronal phenotypes, they are of considerable interest. Thus, efficient methods for identifying novel genes of functional importance in the nervous system, such as cDNA subtraction, remain of great utility. In addition, there can be practical and statistical advantages to focusing on subsets of genes of interest identified by subtractive methods, rather than surveying all genes at once.

## Pitfalls of Subtraction

Many cDNA subtraction techniques are subject to two major problems: (1) the difficulty of identifying low-abundance genes of interest and (2) the tedious screening often necessary to sort through the high number of false positives (background) to find a small number of differentially expressed genes. This latter problem is magnified in the central nervous system owing to the complexity of these tissues and the high number of very low-abundance messages present in the nervous system. These rare but nondifferentially expressed messages often are not subtracted because of the low likelihood of hybridization with their complement in the other subtractive pool.

Several powerful PCR-based techniques for gene discovery that predate microarrays, including differential display PCR (DD-PCR), representational difference analysis (RDA), and suppressive subtractive hybridization (SSH) offered significant improvements over previous subtractive hybridization-based techniques (Lisitsyn and Wigler, 1993; Hubank and Schatz, 1994; Diatchenko et al., 1996). SSH and RDA help to circumvent the problem of background by adding either a normalization step (SSH), or allowing for multiple rounds of subtraction (RDA), with PCR amplification following each subtractive hybridization to reamplify enough material for the next round of subtraction. DD-PCR, although powerful, still suffers from the need to sort through a large background to identify differentially expressed genes (the needle-in-the-haystack problem). This has not been a serious problem using either RDA or SSH in most cases (Hubank and Schatz, 1994; Braun et al., 1995; Diatchenko et al., 1996; O'Neill and Sinclair, 1997; Geschwind et al., 1998b, 2001; Morris et al., 1998; Welford et al., 1998).

## Advantages of Microarrays

Microarrays can be added in series with any subtraction technique to facilitate the differential screening process, similar to the dot blot, or Southern blotting differential screens that are often used (Welford et al., 1998; Yang et al., 1999; Morris et al., 1998). Furthermore, custom-subtracted libraries gridded down as microarrays can be used to monitor gene expression in the specific system of interest. Since these custom-subtracted microarrays assay both known and novel genes, this adds the benefit of studying unknown genes, rather than limiting a study to known genes or ESTs available, which probably account for less than half of the genes expressed in the brain. Further, procurement of large EST libraries is expensive. A custom array made from subtracted clones of interest provides a less expensive route to studying gene expression in a large number of clones of interest. The use of a custom microarray with fewer spots than a genomic-level array also simplifies downstream analysis and statistics. A microarray has the further advantage of cohybridization of both comparison cDNA pools onto the same group of spots, improving reproducibility and facilitating quantitative comparisons. Dynamic range is also improved relative to most radioactive detection methods. Glass slides also have additional advantages over porous, flexible surfaces such as nylon membranes. The high density of spots allows for more efficient probing of a larger number of genes than conventional screening techniques.

One caveat of screening subtracted libraries is that the products of these subtractions are typically about half the size of ESTs, raising the issue of whether these subtracted libraries will perform as well as EST-based libraries containing larger hybridization targets. Currently, in our facility the cost to array 50 slides with 5000 already amplified clones is about $5000, or about $100 per slide. The advantages of microarrays for screening should be balanced against the lower cost of the more standard screening techniques. An additional option to microarrays would be the coupling of RDA or SSH to serial analysis of gene expression (SAGE) to allow the counting of tags to efficiently identify the genes enriched in the subtraction (Welford et al., 1998; Velculescu et al., 1995).

## Microarrays Are an Emerging Technology

cDNA microarray technology is in its infancy and many of its limitations are not well understood, especially with regard to its accuracy and reproducibility. At this point, we view our experiments with microarrays as very efficient exploratory screening experiments that need to be followed by more standard techniques for confirmation of gene expression patterns. We have used a combination of powerful subtraction techniques with microarray technology to study gene expression and to identify novel genes involved in different developmental events in the CNS. In each case we have explored the optimum number of RDA subtraction rounds for each system in order to reach the maximum level of subtraction while preserving the complexity of the mixture, in an attempt to identify the largest number of differentially expressed genes with the lowest background of false positives. These experiments are presented here, one with a simpler mixture of cells and the other with a more complex tissue, as models on which to plan specific experiments in other laboratories.

## Experimental Methods and Results

The basic experimental flow is outlined in table 10.1. Our initial experience with this combination of techniques involved subtraction of the right and left posterior perisylvian region in the developing human fetal brain. SSH and RDA were carried out on homologous samples from the right and left cortex, and the output subtracted libraries were compared on microarrays by differential hybridization with starting amplicons. SSH was done several times but we were unable to obtain clones that were convincingly differentially expressed. This is in contrast to SSH applied to simpler, less complex nervous system tissues and or *in vitro* systems, in which convincing differentially expressed clones have been obtained in numerous cases (e.g., Yang et al., 1999).

Because of the flexibility of the number of rounds, and hence the amount of enrichment that one can obtain with RDA, all of our

**Table 10.1** Experimental scheme

1. Prepare RNA from tissue or cells of interest.

2. Perform RDA subtraction (A-B and B-A). In this case A = NS and B = D.

3. Shotgun clone RDA products to make subtracted libraries.

4. Determine optimal number of rounds for large-scale screening. Screen 100 clones from each round by SAGE, dot blot, or microarray and sequencing of clones to determine degree of differential expression and redundancy.

5. PCR amplify clone inserts from optimal round(s) and array the inserts.

6. Microarray screening

   - Screen with starting A and B amplicons as probe

   and/or

   - Screen with cDNA made directly from A and B mRNA

   and

   - Screen with cDNA from other tissues or cell lines to prioritize further analysis.

7. Partially sequence the highest priority clones to establish their identity.

8. Prioritize clones by homology or novelty.

9. Confirm differential expression (RT-PCR, Northern blotting, or in situ hybridization).

subsequent work has involved RDA. However, for many *in vitro* systems or simple tissues, SSH has the potential to result in a reasonable subtraction and microarray for gene expression studies, provided the smallest products are not arrayed. SSH has the advantage that it is available in a kit form and takes about 1 week to perform (Clontech PCR-Select kit).

**RDA Subtraction**

Typically, RDA is performed as a simultaneous subtraction of two cDNA populations in both directions. One can monitor the progress of the subtraction by observing differences emerging from the two directions of subtraction in successive rounds (figure 10.1). Differentially expressed genes are typically those that are present in one comparison that are not in the reciprocal comparison. Four

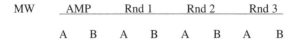

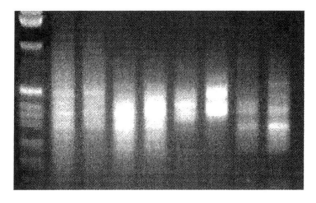

**Figure 10.1** RDA Subtraction. RDA products from each direction of subtraction are separated on a 1.5% agarose gel stained with ethidium bromide. The starting amplicon (AMP) and round of subtraction are marked at the top (Rnd *n*); the direction of subtraction is labeled underneath each round (A = NS and B = D). One can observe the progressive simplification of the products with each round of subtraction until discrete bands are visible on the gel in round 3.

rounds of RDA can yield a several millionfold amplification of differentially expressed sequences. Thus, RDA has been used successfully to identify the differential presence of single-copy regions from genomic DNA and complex populations of cDNA. Further, RDA has been shown to readily identify low abundance (1 to 10 copies per cell) that is expressed in 1% of cells in a heterogeneous mixture (Hubank and Shatz, 1994).

Several published papers present details of RDA subtraction, including the original paper by Hubank and Shatz (1994) adapting genomic RDA to cDNA. We use a protocol based on Hubank and Shatz (1994) and modified by others (Nelson and Denny, 1999; Welford et al., 1998; O'Neill and Sinclair, 1997; Braun et al., 1995; Geschwind et al., 2001). Figure 10.1 depicts the relative enrichment of differentially expressed products that one can expect as RDA progresses. This RDA was carried out with neurosphere cultures containing neural progenitors before (NS) and after (D) a differentiation stimulus. Genes expressed in the NS-D subtraction might represent markers for neural progenitor cells at various stages of commitment. Typically, an RDA subtraction would proceed to four rounds and the differentially expressed bands would be isolated from the gel. Instead, we shotgun clone each round and array a small random sample of the subtracted libraries to determine the optimum number of rounds to subject to a large-scale microarray screen. With this screening protocol, it is seldom necessary to complete all four rounds, and often two rounds are enough, saving time relative to conventional RDA. The RDA takes 2 weeks, followed by a few days for subcloning subtracted libraries.

It is easy to introduce artifacts in any microarray or PCR-based subtraction experiment, a problem magnified when the techniques are coupled. Thus, we use ART tips and store RDA reagents separately. We have adapted the modifications introduced by others to the original RDA protocol (see Welford et al., 1998; O'Neill and Sinclair, 1997). Details of this protocol have been published (Nelson and Denny, 1999). The RDA protocol can be obtained on our website at http://geschwindlab.medsch.ucla.edu. We have made the following additional modifications: (1) Tester to driver ratios are decreased for round 1 to 1:40; for round 2 to 1:400; for round 3 to 1:4000; for round 4 to 1:20,000. (2) Primers and adapters are HPLC purified (O'Neill and Sinclair, 1997). (3) Amplicons are purified from adaptors most effectively using the microcon-100 spin concentrator (Millipore), rather than Qiagen columns or other more cumbersome methods, such as gel purification.

**Microarray Screen**

SHOTGUN CLONING AND ARRAYING
Subtracted cDNA is DpnII digested and shotgun cloned into the BamH1 site of pBluescript. These subtracted libraries are plated out and the clones are randomly picked into 96 well plates for ar-

raying, where they are grown overnight. To amplify clone inserts, a small volume of the culture is added to a PCR reaction mixture with amido-modified, or nonmodified vector-specific primers. Amplified clone inserts from the PCR reactions are ethanol precipitated and resuspended in 8 to 10 μl of 350 mM, pH 9.0 sodium bicarbonate arraying buffer for a final concentration of 400–1000 ng/μl. Each clone insert is checked on a gel for purity and size prior to arraying. It takes two people about 2 to 4 weeks to prepare and array 2000–5000 clones, including allowance for mistakes. This will vary, depending on the laboratories' PCR throughput and available staff. Arraying onto poly-L-lysine-coated slides and hybridization is done essentially according to the Brown lab protocols (see the appendix at the end of this volume for an address). One difficulty we have encountered using quill tips for arraying is variability, which is usually due to tip wobble or wear. Arrayers that use non-quill-based designs may provide more reproducible arrays, although this remains to be demonstrated.

The following minor modifications have been made: Following hybridization, two 5-minute washes, 2× SSC and 0.1% SDS and 0.2× SSC are used. Twenty to thirty micrograms of human $C_0t$-1 DNA are used to block nonspecific hybridization. Optimal probe labeling is accomplished with overnight random primer labeling.

**Protocol**   Probe labeling

> Probes are labeled using Stratagene "Prime-It" random primer-labeling kit. Follow the manufacturer's instructions for random hexamer labeling using 10 U Klenow exo-polymerase per reaction with the following modifications: (1) To maximize label incorporation, reduce dCTP to 50 μM; dope dCTP-Cy3 or Cy5 in to 60 μM and (2) conduct labeling overnight for 12 to 16 hours. Probes are mixed together with 20 μg mouse $C_0t$ 1 DNA (Gibco 18440-016), ethanol precipitated and resuspended in 20 μl hybridization buffer. Hybridization buffer: 3.5 × SSC, 2.5 Denhardt's solution, 0.1% SDS. For other protocols, see our website, http://geschwindlab.medsch.ucla.edu.

In figure 10.2 (see also plate 8), round 2 RDA products in both directions of subtraction (NS-D and D-NS) were randomly picked after plating at low density. The inserts were PCR amplified with vector-specific primers flanking the inserts, ethanol precipitated, and resuspended in arraying buffer in 96 well plates at a DNA concentration of between 400 and 1000 ng/μl. These amplified inserts from randomly chosen clones were arrayed using the Cartesian microarrayer at a spacing of about 300 μM (4-pin configuration). The average clone insert size is about 500 bp.

These arrays were probed by cohybridization with differentially labeled (Cy3 or Cy5) starting amplicons, as shown to the right of the arrays. The two groups of $8 \times 6$ spots in each array are duplicates, and the top and bottom arrays are also duplicates of each other, but the probes have been labeled with different fluors. The slides were scanned with a custom-built confocal scanning laser microscope (built by Stan Nelson and John Parker, UCLA School of Medicine). Currently we use commercial scanners that appear to have a high sensitivity. Cy3 and Cy5 spots are normalized to control spots printed in each quadrant (G3PDH). Noneukaryotic genes and plasmids without inserts are arrayed as negative controls. The images are false color overlays (Cy5 = red, Cy3 = green) derived from images analyzed with the ImaGene software package (Bio-Discovery). Spots labeled C1, E1, and G3 highlight a few of the differentially expressed clones in the NS-D direction.

Several points should be made with regard to screening this subtraction with microarrays:

- The array hybridizations appear to be reproducible; most clones that show the maximal degree of differential expression in one hybridization do so in another. The coefficient of variation ranges between 4 and 13% for duplicate or multiply redundant spots on the same array.

It may also be valuable to compare control or experimental conditions with each other to define the system's variability and reproducibility of hybridization signals. One such comparison is

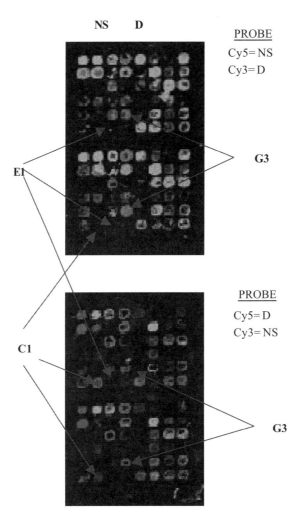

**Figure 10.2** Magnified microarray quadrants. Magnified false color images of a pilot microarray of RDA round 2 subtraction products. Clones from the NS-D direction are arrayed in the first four columns on the left side of the array under NS, and those from the D-NS direction are arrayed in columns 5–6 on the right under D. Both arrays shown are duplicates of each other, with the labeling dyes switched to indicate that the differential labeling represents differential hybridization and is not an artifact of the probe label. See plate 8 for color version.

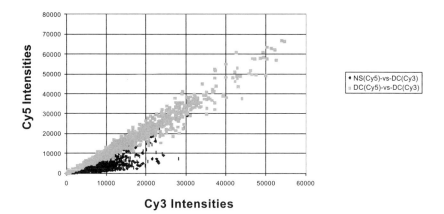

**Cy3 Intensities**

**Figure 10.3**  Data quality and visualization. cDNA from the DC condition was labeled with Cy3 and Cy5 and cohybridized onto an array with 960 D enriched elements and 2280 NS enriched elements. Hybridizations to the D spots are labeled as light gray boxes (control hybridization). An experimental hybridization to identify clones enriched in the NS condition is graphed as black diamonds. The vast majority of data points from the control hybridization fall close to the line with a slope of 1.0, whereas in the experimental condition, most clones fall off this line, demonstrating significant differential expression. In each experiment, Cy3 and Cy5 intensity has been normalized using G3PDH. Intensities are represented as absolute values of integrated intensities at each clone.

presented in figure 10.3. cDNA from the same DC populations were each labeled with Cy3 and Cy5 and cohybridized onto the array. If hybridizations were perfectly invariate and reproducible, graphing Cy3 and Cy5 signals for all array elements would yield a line with a slope of 1.0 and correlation of 1.0. The slope in this particular experiment was 1.08 and $r = 0.98$, indicating very consistent hybridizations.

- All clones differentially expressed on the array that have been tested with Northern blotting show a similar magnitude and direction of differential expression ($n = 20$), as has been observed in simpler non-neural culture systems (Welford et al., 1998). After two rounds of subtraction in the neurosphere experiment (representative of in vitro systems), approximately 60% of the clones are differentially expressed in the proper direction (ratio > 1.0) and 25% demonstrate twofold or greater differential expression.

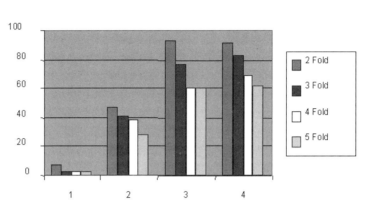

**RDA Round Number**

**Figure 10.4** Progressive enrichment by RDA round. The percentage of clones with *n*-fold differential expression in the left minus right posterior superior temporal gyrus (STG); subtraction is depicted for each round of RDA. More than half of the clones enriched by RDA show a fivefold or greater ratio of differential expression by round 3. Between three and four rounds of RDA, it appears as if a plateau is reached.

- Genes with known roles in this system, or known to be differentially expressed, comprise some of the clones that we have identified as differentially expressed using this screen, confirming the biological relevance of the changes observed in gene expression.
- In cases where the relative abundance of a gene product is known or can be estimated, the amount of signal is correlated with the abundance of a given mRNA.

How many rounds of RDA are optimal for a given system? The percentage of clones that are differentially expressed increases with each round of RDA, as depicted in figure 10.4. Although this graph shows that the percentage of clones with a given degree of differential expression increases in each successive round of RDA, it does not show that the complexity of the libraries decreases in tandem. Since the goal is to exhaustively screen the subtracted library containing the largest number of unique, differentially expressed clones, not necessarily the library containing the largest percentage of differentially expressed clones, it helps to have some measure of redundancy of the subtracted library.

**Table 10.2** Clone redundancy and novelty

|  | ROUND 1 | ROUND 2 | ROUND 3 | ROUND 4 |
|---|---|---|---|---|
| STG |  |  |  |  |
| Percent duplicates |  | 5–8 | 42–44 | 54–83 |
| Percent novel genes |  | 45 | 26 | 25 |
| Neurospheres |  |  |  |  |
| Percent duplicates |  | 28 | 69 | NA |
| Percent novel genes |  | 50 | 18 | NA |

*Notes:* NA, Not applicable.

We have sequenced a random sample of differentially expressed clones from each round to determine redundancy. The data are presented in table 10.2 for a complex tissue (superior temporal gyrus, STG) and a simpler system (neurospheres).

Although in the STG subtraction, round 2 has low redundancy and a high number of clones representing novel genes, the percentage of clones that are differentially expressed more than five-fold is less than 25%, while in round 3, 60% of the clones show a fivefold or greater differential expression (figure 10.4). Thus it appears as if three rounds are optimal for yielding the largest percentage of novel clones showing significant differential expression. If a cell culture system or simple tissue is to be used, two rounds are likely to be optimal. However, this may vary in a given system. One can determine the complexity of the subtracted library by doing a small-scale dot blot or microarray (e.g., figure 10.1) at each level of subtraction or assay a small number of randomly picked clones at each level of subtraction as shown earlier. Once the optimum RDA round for screening is identified, a large number of clones from that round can be arrayed at high density and screened by differential hybridization. One should determine library titer and sequence a subset of differentially expressed clones prior to arraying, so as not to oversaturate the array with redundant clones.

If some clones are known genes, they can be used to monitor the expression experiments.

## Secondary Screening

PRIORITIZATION OF CLONES FOR FURTHER STUDY
After the initial array probing, the number of clones to be analyzed further depends upon the type of downstream analysis necessary to confirm differential expression. If sequencing is available and inexpensive, it may be possible to sequence all differentially expressed clones on a given array. In the case where downstream analysis may be more tedious, one can focus on those clones showing changes in expression in the top 20%, or 3% of arrayed clones, for example (slightly more than one and two standard deviations above the mean change, respectively).

Alternatively, one can further prioritize clones by studying their expression patterns in subsequent array experiments. For example, one can probe the array with cDNA from a number of neural and non-neural tissues from different developmental stages to rapidly focus on the set of genes that are nervous system enriched and stage specific. In addition, one can focus on those spots with the lowest hybridization signals because these typically represent the most unique clones. Signal strength depends upon abundance of the cDNA in the probe since more abundant genes give stronger signals.

A typical screening procedure involves: (1) screening 2000–5000 clones by microarray; (2) sequencing and performing homology searching and alignments on the top group of clones (typically 16% = 1 SD); (3) prioritization by homology or novelty; and (4) Northern blotting or in situ hybridization to confirm differential expression.

OTHER SCREENING CONSIDERATIONS
Some commonsense recommendations for secondary screening are to: (1) identify a source for relatively low-cost single-pass sequencing of differentially expressed clones and (2) identify RNA sources

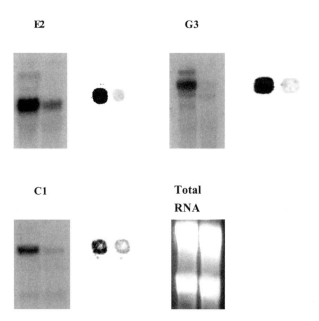

**Figure 10.5** Northern blot confirmation of array data. Array spots are depicted alongside Northern blots of NS (left) and D (right) RNA for three different clones: E2, G3, and C1. Total RNA is shown in the bottom right of the figure as a loading control, and GP3DH is used as a final control for hybridization (not shown); some slight distortions of the spots have occurred during cutting and pasting of the figure.

or amplification methods that permit complete, efficient screening. Several techniques for amplification of cDNA permit the use of small pieces of tissue or single cells (Eberwine et al., 1992; Eberwine, 1996; see also chapters 8 and 9 in this volume; Clontech "SMART cDNA kit"). Owing to the scarcity of tissue, we have chosen to use sequencing, followed by RT-PCR and in situ hybridization to screen the left and right STG subtraction. For the neurosphere subtraction, we have used Northern blotting and in situ hybridization as secondary confirmation following sequencing (Geschwind et al., 2001). Using the Ambion EZ strip procedure, we have been able to re-use blots at least five times to detect low-abundance species. Three representative Northern blots confirming the differential expression of C1 and G3 are shown in figure 10.5 as an example of secondary screening.

Are subtracted arrays as useful for gene expression studies as EST or other clone-based arrays? Although subtracted arrays will enrich for clones of interest and allow the study of novel genes, the average insert size of arrayed clones obtained from the usual PCR-based subtractions is about half the size of commercially available cDNA clones (300 to 600 bp versus 1.2 kb for ESTs). Unfortunately, there has been no published direct comparison of these subtraction-based arrays with larger insert clone-based arrays.

Several commercially available and custom microarrays (e.g., M. Potier, chapter 9) rely on small PCR-amplified fragments of genes and appear reliable, as do oligonucleotide arrays. Our experience with these subtracted arrays has been that duplicates on the same array show similar hybridization patterns, but that between hybridizations there can be some variability in absolute hybridization onto the array. Depending on the method of normalization used, spots that are in the top 10 to 20% of differential regulation in one array are very likely to be in the same range in a duplicate hybridization, suggesting reasonable reproducibility. The coefficient of variance is also usually lower than 20%. We have demonstrated that the quality of the data in terms of variability of cohybridized duplicate amplicons obtained from the subtracted array is high. Experiments using a generic mouse 9K array indicate that about one-half of the genes that we detected using the custom array were not present on the generic array, demonstrating the utility of the subtraction-based approach.

So far, those clones demonstrating significant differential hybridization on microarrays almost always demonstrate differential hybridization on Northern blot analysis (Geschwind et al., 2001; Terskikh et al., 2001). However, the precise value of differential hybridization does not always match, whether the array is EST based, or otherwise. Typically this reflects compression of the ratios on arrays relative to Northern blots, which may be due to the lower stringency array hybridizations that result in higher background. Currently, it is prudent to take the position that crucial quantitative data based on microarray-based hybridizations should be confirmed with more conventional techniques.

## Summary and Conclusions

A large number of novel, differentially expressed genes can be detected using microarrays to screen the products of RDA or other cDNA subtractions. The coupling of these subtraction techniques with cDNA microarrays offers neuroscientists increased power to study gene regulation in complex CNS tissues. The advantages of using subtracted libraries for microarray screening include the ability to use less starting RNA for probing than on commercial arrays, the ability to identify and characterize novel genes, and the ability to focus the analysis on genes of specific interest without a priori biases. Once a subtracted array is made, it may also be useful as a tool for studying gene expression in other related biological systems (Geschwind et al., 2001; Terskikh et al., 2001). The combination of this method in tandem with other high-resolution anatomical techniques, such as laser capture microdissection or single-cell PCR, offers the promise of unprecedented ability to study gene expression in the nervous system.

## Acknowledgments

This work was partially supported by the National Institutes of Health (grant NS01849, National Institute of Neurological Disorders and Stroke; grant MH60233, National Institute of Mental Health), and the Ron Shapiro Charitable Foundation. DG is grateful to his collaborator Harley Kornblum (neurosphere project) and to Christopher Denny for guiding me through our first RDA experiment.

## References

Braun BS, Frieden R, Lessnick SL, May WA, and Denny CT (1995). Identification of target genes for the Ewing's sarcoma EWS/FLI fusion protein by representational difference analysis. *Mol Cell Biol* 15: 4623–30.

DeRisi J, Penland L, Brown PO, Bittner ML, Meltzer PS, Ray M, and Chen Y et al. (1996). Use of a cDNA microarray to analyze gene expression patterns in human cancer. *Nat Genet* 14: 457–60.

Diatchenko L, Lau YF, Campbell AP, Chenchik A, Moqadam F, Huang B, and Lukyanov S et al. (1996). Suppression subtractive hybridization: A method for generating differentially regulated or tissue-specific cDNA probes and libraries. *Proc Natl Acad Sci USA* 93: 6025–30.

Eberwine J (1996). Amplification of mRNA populations using aRNA generated from immobilized oligo(dT)-T7 primed cDNA. *Biotechniques* 20: 584–91.

Eberwine J, Yeh H, Miyashiro K, Cao Y, Nair S, Finnell R, Zettel M, and Coleman P (1992). Analysis of gene expression in single live neurons. *Proc Natl Acad Sci USA* 89: 3010–14.

Geschwind DH, Gregg J, Boone K, Karrim J, Pawlikowska-Haddal A, Rao E, Ellison J, Ciccodicola A, D'Urso M, Woods R, Rappold GA, Swerdloff R, and Nelson SF (1998a). Klinefelter's syndrome as a model of anomalous cerebral laterality: Testing gene dosage in the X chromosome pseudoautosomal region using a DNA microarray. *Dev Genet* 23: 215–29.

Geschwind DH, Loginov M, Karrim J, and Nelson SF (1998b). Finding the differences between the developing cerebral hemispheres using RDA and DNA microarray technology. *Society for Neuroscience Abstracts* 24(1): 398.3.

Geschwind DH, Ou J, Easterday MC, Dougherty JD, Jackson RJ, Chen Z, Antoine H, Terskikh A, Weissman IL, Nelson SF, and Kornblum HI (2001). A genetic analysis of neural progenitor differentiation. *Neuron* 29: 325–39.

Hubank M and Schatz DG (1994). Identifying differences in mRNA expression by representational difference analysis of cDNA. *Nucleic Acids Res* 22: 5640–8.

Lisitsyn N and Wigler M (1993). Cloning the differences between two complex genomes. *Science* 259: 946–51.

Morris ME, Viswanathan N, Kuhlman S, Davis FC, and Weitz CJ (1998). A screen for genes induced in the suprachiasmatic nucleus by light. *Science* 279: 1544–7.

Nelson SF and Denny C (1999). Representational differences analysis and microarray hybridization for efficient cloning and screening of differentially expressed genes. In *DNA Microarrays: A Practical Approach*. Mark Schena, ed., Oxford University Press, New York, pp. 43–58.

O'Neill MJ and Sinclair AH (1997). Isolation of rare transcripts by representational difference analysis. *Nucleic Acids Res* 25: 2681–2.

Schena M, Shalon D, Davis RW, and Brown PO (1995). Quantitative monitoring of gene expression patterns with a complementary DNA microarray. *Science* 270: 467–70.

Shalon D, Smith SJ, and Brown PO (1996). A DNA microarray system for analyzing complex DNA samples using two-color fluorescent probe hybridization. *Genome Res* 6: 639–45.

Terskikh AV, Easterday MC, Li L, Hood L, Kornblum HI, Geschwind DH, and Weissman IL (2001). From hematopoiesis to neuropoiesis: Evidence of overlapping genetic programs. *Proc Natl Acad Sci USA* 98: 7934–9.

Velculescu VE, Zhang L, Vogelstein B, and Kinzler KW (1995). Serial analysis of gene expression. *Science* 270: 484–7.

Welford SM, Gregg J, Chen E, Garrison D, Sorensen PH, Denny CT, and Nelson SF (1998). Detection of differentially expressed genes in primary tumor tissues using representational differences analysis coupled to microarray hybridization. *Nucleic Acids Res* 26: 3059–65.

Yang GP, Ross DT, Kuang WW, Brown PO, and Weigel RJ (1999). Combining SSH and cDNA microarrays for rapid identification of differentially expressed genes. *Nucleic Acids Res* 27: 1517–23.

# 11 Tracing Genetic Information Flow from Gene Expression to Pathways and Regulatory Networks

*Stefanie Fuhrman, Patrik D'haeseleer, Shoudan Liang, and Roland Somogyi*

Novel, high-throughput technologies are opening global perspectives on living organisms at the molecular level. Together with a vast experimental literature on biomolecular processes, these data are now providing researchers with the challenge of multifunctionality, implying the existence of molecular networks as opposed to isolated, linear pathways of causality. Questions that have traditionally been posed in the singular are now being addressed in the plural:

- What are the sequences of all of the genes on this genome?
- Where are the active sites of this protein?
- What are the functions of this gene?
- Which genes regulate this gene?
- Which genes are responsible for this disease?
- Which drugs will cure this disease?

Beginning with gene sequencing, the structures of tens of thousands of genes are being identified, along with a variety of structural and regulatory features that provide functional clues. However, only the molecular machinery of the cell is able to consistently translate the sequence information into the functions that determine the complex genetic and biochemical networks that define the behavior of an organism. Since we ultimately seek understanding of the regulatory skeleton of these networks, we are also taking steps to monitor their molecular activities on a global level to reflect the effective functional state of a biological system. Several technologies (such as hybridization microarrays, automated RT-PCR, 2D gel electrophoresis, and antibody arrays) allow the assaying of RNA and the elucidating of protein expression profiles with differing levels of precision and depth.

How should this process of acquiring activity data be organized, and how should these results be interpreted in order to find therapeutic targets and critical processes for bioengineering? Here it is crucial to find the proper abstractions around which to build modeling frameworks and data analysis tools. These abstractions must be centered around two important principles:

- *Genetic information flow: Defining the mapping from sequence space to functional space.* Clearly, the genome contains the information for constructing the complex molecular features of an organism, as reflected in the process of development. In information terms, the complexity of the fully developed organism cannot be higher than that of the genome. Which processes link these two types of information? In other words, what are the codes that translate sequence into structure and function? We are looking for representations of these codes in a form understandable to us, so that we may apply them to model building and prediction. We therefore seek methods that allow us to extract these codes from gene sequence and activity data.

- *Complex dynamic systems: From states to trajectories to attractors.* When addressing biological function, we usually refer to functions in time (i.e., causality and dynamics). On a molecular level, function is manifested in the action of complex networks. The dynamics of these networks resemble trajectories of state transitions; this is what we are monitoring when conducting temporal gene expression surveys. The concept of attractors is what really lends meaning to these trajectories; that is, the attractors are the high-dimensional dynamic molecular representations of stable phenotypic structures such as differentiated cells or tissues—healthy or diseased (Kauffman, 1993; Somogyi and Sniegoski, 1996).

The goal of investigators is to understand the dynamics to the point where they can predict the attractor of a molecular network and know enough about the network architecture to direct these networks to attractors of choice (i.e., from a cancerous cell type to a benign cell type, from degeneration to regeneration).

This chapter focuses on tools that allow the discovery and integration of gene function in the context of large-scale gene expression data. This approach is particularly important to the neurosciences, since the nervous system involves the integration of many molecular species originating from inter- and intracellular signaling gene families. Measurement, analysis, and inference can be conducted at several levels, ranging from simple comparisons to the clustering of genes into pathways to the reverse engineering of critical causal molecular connections.

## Comparative Analysis of Microarray Data

A key mission of neuroscience research is to identify the molecular basis of neurological disorders through the study of disease models. The value of a model system for disorders depends on two principal characteristics: (1) it must be experimentally accessible and (2) it must reproduce relevant aspects of a disease phenotype. Cell cultures and animal models meet the criterion of accessibility, but there is much room for improvement in demonstrating their phenotypic relevance to human disease. Large-scale gene expression surveys offer a new, in-depth means to assign a phenotype to cells and animals used as research tools for disease.

Initial studies demonstrate the power of microarray and large-scale RT-PCR methods in isolating patterns of gene expression that are characteristic of mouse stem cell differentiation models and rat brain injury (see later discussion). Retinoic acid was used to differentiate mouse embryonic stem (ES) cells into neurons (J. F. Loring, unpublished results). A competitive expression survey was carried out with the mouse GEM1 microarray of public domain genes and expressed sequence tags, covering 8700 clones (http://www.incyte.com/products/arrays/pdgems.html).

Differential expression responses for four different RNA samples (differentiated and control cultures) can be captured in a dot-plot format, each point mapping the expression ratios for an individual gene (figure 11.1). Most points on the horizontal scale (control cul-

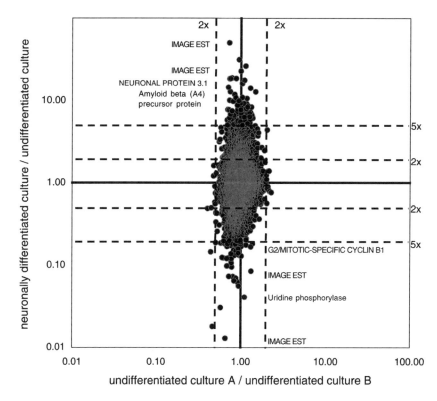

**Figure 11.1** Analysis of a microarray survey of mouse stem cell differentiation. Differential expression of genes is shown on a range from 100-fold downregulation (0.01) to 100-fold upregulation; twofold and fivefold differential expression guides are shown as broken lines. The horizontal axis shows expression ratios for a competitive hybridization of two independent, undifferentiated control cultures (each point resembles a gene). The vertical axis shows expression ratios for a neuronally differentiated culture vs. an undifferentiated culture (points on the upper half of the graph correspond to genes induced during neuronal differentiation). (Data analysis courtesy of Jeanne F. Loring.)

ture comparison) cluster close to a differential expression value of 1.00, and generally within the twofold limit. This demonstrates that there is little background fluctuation among ES cell lines while they remain undifferentiated. However, competitive hybridization of RNA from neuronally differentiated cells to RNA from a control culture reveals a wide vertical spread of differential expression (94 genes upregulated $\geq$ fivefold; 62 genes downregulated $\geq$ fivefold). Note the upregulation of two known neuronal marker genes and the downregulation of cell division-related genes, as expected for this model.

By also identifying ESTs in the strongly differentially expressed set, we are providing the first functional clues for these novel genes. Databases of profiles such as those shown in the example may help categorize the signatures of many healthy and diseased cell types, providing a tool for diagnostic categorization and therapeutic target selection.

### Prioritizing Genes According to Expression Diversity (Shannon Entropy)

One analytical method now being widely considered in functional genomics is clustering (see later discussion). Clustering is the grouping of genes according to similarities in their temporal or anatomical expression patterns. Clustering provides clues to possible shared functions among genes that have not previously been associated.

Another type of method was introduced by Fuhrman and colleagues (2000) and involves the use of Shannon entropy (Shannon and Weaver, 1963)—an information theoretic measure—to select putative drug targets from among thousands of genes expressed in parallel.

Shannon entropy is defined as

$$H = -\sum p_i \log_2(p_i)$$

where $p_i$ is the probability (frequency) of a level of expression of a gene. This concept should not be confused with disorder or randomness. Shannon entropy is a measure of the information content of a dynamic pattern—in this case a time series of gene expression. The greater the variation or change in a pattern, the higher the entropy. Figure 11.2 provides a detailed explanation.

As shown in the figure, changes in gene expression can be measured using Shannon entropy. Change or variation in gene expression is also the criterion used by biologists in determining which genes are physiologically relevant to the biological process being studied. Genes whose expression levels change in response to a disease or perturbation are logical candidates for drug targets, since these are the genes that actively participate in the disease process. It is for this reason that the use of Shannon entropy to select drug target candidates was proposed (Fuhrman et al., 2000).

When dealing with thousands of genes—all potential drug targets—it is desirable to order the genes according to their degree of participation in a physiological process. Genes with the highest Shannon entropy can therefore be selected out as likely drug target candidates, permitting pharmaceutical scientists to focus their efforts and limited resources on those genes.

Shannon entropy may also be used as a measure of anatomical complexity in the CNS (Fuhrman et al., 2000) by substituting brain regions for time points (see figure 11.3 for a complete explanation). Genes that are differentially expressed over a set of brain regions may be considered important contributors to the complexity of brain anatomy, whereas those that show no differences in expression across the brain are of less interest. This is reminiscent of part of the definition of a neurotransmitter—a substance that is differentially distributed. Otherwise, water could be considered a neurotransmitter. Like water, genes that exhibit no anatomical differences in expression may be regarded as the milieu in which other genes operate. The same can be said for temporal patterns. Genes that show no changes in expression over time are likely to be running in the background; they may be necessary for life, but will not allow us to distinguish among the different physiological processes being studied.

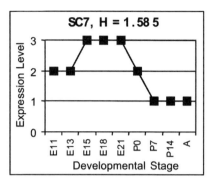
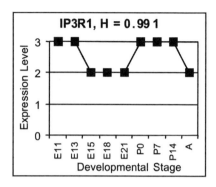
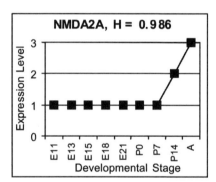
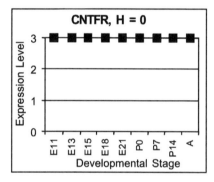

**Figure 11.2** Gene expression time series from developing rat spinal cord (data from Wen et al., 1998). With nine time points (embryonic day 11 to postnatal day 90) and three levels of gene expression, Shannon entropy (H) ranges from 0 to 1.585. The ciliary neurotrophic factor receptor (CNTFR) has zero entropy because its expression pattern is invariant over time. SC7 (an EST) has the highest possible entropy for nine time points and three expression levels, since its pattern varies over time and the expression levels are spread out as much as possible (three data points at each of three expression levels). $N$-Methyl-D-aspartate receptor 2A (NMDA2A) exhibits all three expression levels, but most of the pattern is at one level, so this gene has submaximal entropy. Inositol trisphosphate receptor 1 (IP3R1) exhibits only two out of three expression levels, and so has submaximal entropy. It has been demonstrated that the number of expression level bins for these calculations should be less than or equal to the $\log_2$ of the number of events (Bruce Sawhill, unpublished observations). For fewer than 8 time points, 2 bins may be used; for 8 or more time points, 3 bins; for 16 or more, 4 bins, etc.

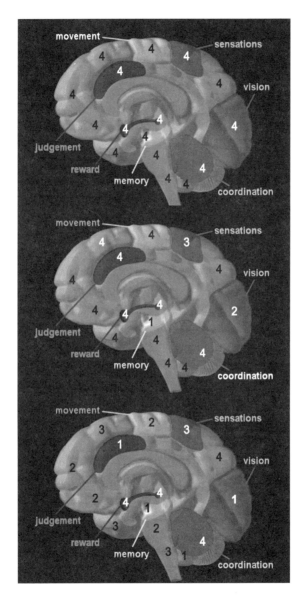

**Figure 11.3** Hypothetical gene expression patterns given four levels of expression at a single time point. Top panel: A gene that is expressed at the same level in each of 16 brain regions has zero information content ($H = 0$). Middle panel: This gene is expressed at the same level in most regions assayed ($H = 0.99$). Bottom panel: Expression at all

We have applied Shannon entropy to several data sets (Fuhrman et al., 2000): developing rat spinal cord (112 genes, 9 time points); developing rat hippocampus and hippocampus after a kainate-induced seizure (70 genes, 11 time points; unpublished observations); and rat liver after exposure to toxic doses of several compounds (1000 genes, 7 time points; unpublished observations).

The spinal cord and liver results suggest that certain functional groups are overrepresented at high entropy values. For example, in the developing spinal cord, neurotransmitter receptor and neurotransmitter metabolizing enzyme genes are enriched at the highest entropy values. Similarly, in liver, flavoproteins (among other groups) are enriched at the highest entropy value in response to toxic doses of clofibrate or acetaminophen; hexosyl transferases and other groups are overrepresented at high entropy in response to a toxic dose of benzo(a)pyrene. This encourages the assaying of other genes from these groups because they appear to be major participants in spinal cord development and hepatotoxicity, respectively.

Specific genes with high Shannon entropy may be selected out for further study as possible drug targets. For example, in post-seizure hippocampus (a model of temporal lobe epilepsy), we find that certain neurotransmitter receptor genes have high entropy: 5HT3 (ionotropic serotonin receptor), GABA-A receptor $\beta$3 subunit, 5HT2 and 5HT1B (metabotropic serotonin receptors), nicotinic receptor $\alpha$3 subunit (ionotropic cholinergic receptor), and mGluR8 (metabotropic glutamate receptor). These receptors are logical choices as drug target candidates for the temporal lobe epilepsy model. Given their genes' high entropy after kainate-induced seizure, it would be worth testing agonists and antagonists for these receptors to determine whether they have any effects on the seizure-related pathology.

four levels with each level equally represented contains the highest level of information content possible with four expression levels and 16 regions ($H = 2.00$). This gene may be said to contribute more to the complexity of brain anatomy than the two genes represented in the top and middle panels.

Both clustering and entropy are well suited to the analysis of long-term events involving multiple genes. In future studies of tissue degeneration and regeneration, it may be beneficial to combine these data analysis methods. For example, entropy could be used to identify possible drug targets in a rat spinal cord regeneration model. The most active regeneration-specific genes could be selected out in this manner. These could then be clustered with genes from a control for normal development. In this way it would be possible to identify development-related genes that act in concert with regeneration-specific genes during the regeneration process.

To summarize, studies of complex processes such as degeneration and regeneration must be designed to account for the lengths of time and numbers of genes involved. The first step is the design of experiments based on the timing of the process, including the interval length and total time course, as well as the selection of genes to be assayed. Next, the appropriate computational methods should be applied to organize the data into an intelligible form. This approach should promote the development of effective treatments for degenerative diseases, such as Alzheimer's disease, and the regeneration of tissue after stroke or injury.

### Inference of Pathways from Cluster Analysis of Time Series

A more in-depth analysis of gene function requires diverse sets of expression data—such as time series of gene expression following a natural or induced response. One of the most revealing natural processes for the examination of gene function is development, in which the differentiation of many cell types can be observed through the action of a complex genetic signaling network. We have used a high-precision RT-PCR method to measure the expression of 70 genes in hippocampal development (figure 11.4). The lower detection limit of ten molecules per sample, and a dynamic range spanning six to eight orders of magnitude of this method, assures us that we will not miss any important fluctuations in gene expression, even for signaling genes, which are often expressed at low but physiologically relevant levels.

The second level of analysis should be focused on classifying the gene expression patterns into similar groups and assessing these groups in terms of functional pathways. Several methods will be illustrated here, each with its own advantages and disadvantages. All of these methods depend on the definition of a similarity measure between individual expression patterns. We have chosen the Euclidean distance, which is simply the distance between two points in an $n$-dimensional Euclidean space, $n$ being the number of measurements conducted—i.e.,

$$D = \sqrt{\left[\sum (A_i - B_i)^2\right]}$$

$A$ and $B$ being the genes and $i$ being the measurement points. This similarity measure is used to compute all the gene-to-gene distances, and the results are stored in a distance matrix.

One of the most intuitive methods for grouping these data sets is agglomerative clustering using the centroid method. This algorithm simply identifies the smallest distance in the distance matrix, joins this gene pair, and replaces the individual genes with the newly defined cluster centroid. The distance matrix is updated with the new centroid data point, and the next minimal distance is identified for the next pairwise joining step. The output of this procedure is a dendrogram that reflects all the joining events, as well as the level of similarity at which the joins took place.

In figures 11.4A and B we show the resulting arrangement of gene expression patterns, with the bifurcation tree shown on the left. The tree has been divided into 20 evenly spaced discrete levels of depth; therefore, the location of each gene can be described by a simple 20-digit numerical classifier.

In order to define the clusters, the tree has to be "pruned" at a user-chosen level of depth. In figure 11.4A, the similarity tree was cut at level three, resulting in 8 remaining clusters; in figure 11.4B, it was cut at level five, resulting in 16 clusters. The difference between these two groupings lies in the method of normalization. The data were normalized to mininum = 0 and maximum = 1 for figure 11.4A and maximum = 1 for figure 11.4B. For agglomerative

**A**

| Cluster bifurcation | Gene | E15 E18 P0 P3 P7 P10 P14 P21 A | Cis-element | Cluster no. |
|---|---|---|---|---|
| | cyclinA | | | 1 |
| | cyclinB | | | 1 |
| | G67I8086 | | | 1 |
| | G67I86 | | | 1 |
| | Brm | | | 1 |
| | nestin | | | 1 |
| | IGFR2 | | | 1 |
| | IGFR1 | | | 1 |
| | H4 | | | 1 |
| | ODC | | | 1 |
| | IGF2 | | | 1 |
| | GAD65 | | | 1 |
| | GRg3 | | | 1 |
| | GRa3 | | | 1 |
| | actin | | | 1 |
| | cellubrevin | | | 1 |
| | GRg2 | | | 1 |
| | IP3R3 | | | 1 |
| | 5HT3 | | | 1 |
| | TCP | | | 1 |
| | EGF | | | 1 |
| | GRa5 | | | 2 |
| | GRa1 | | | 2 |
| | IP3R2 | | | 2 |
| | S100beta | | | 2 |
| | NFL | | Krox-24 | 2 |
| | nAChRa5 | | | 2 |
| | mGluR3 | | | 2 |
| | GRa4 | | | 2 |
| | NT3 | | | 2 |
| | GRb1 | | | 2 |
| | GAD67 | | Krox-24 | 2 |
| | GRa2 | | | 2 |
| | GRg1 | | | 2 |
| | 5HT1b | | | 2 |
| | NFM | | | 2 |
| | bFGF | | Krox-24 | 2 |
| | GFAP | | | 2 |
| | mAChR2 | | | 2 |
| | GRb2 | | | 2 |
| | nAChRa7 | | Krox-24 | 2 |
| | preGAD67 | | | 2 |
| | NFH | | | 2 |
| | synaptophysin | | | 2 |
| | FABP | | | 2 |
| | PDGFb | | | 2 |
| | PDGFR | | | 2 |
| | GRb3 | | | 2 |
| | mAChR1 | | | 2 |
| | ACHE | | Krox-24 | 2 |
| | mGluR8 | | | 2 |
| | 5HT2 | | | 2 |
| | CX43 | | | 2 |
| | neno | | Krox-24 | 2 |
| | IGF1 | | | 2 |
| | aFGF | | | 3 |
| | GAP43 | | | 4 |
| | CCO1 | | | 5 |
| | MOG | | | 6 |
| | cjun | | | 6 |
| | BDNF | | | 6 |
| | MK2 | | | 7 |
| | CCO2 | | | 7 |
| | TH | | | 7 |
| | CNTF | | | 7 |
| | CNTFR | | | 7 |
| | GMFb | | | 7 |
| | nAChRa3 | | | 8 |
| | InsR | | | 8 |
| | trkC | | | 8 |

**B**

| Cluster bifurcation | Gene | E15 E18 P0 P3 P7 P10 P14 P21 A | Cis-element | Cluster no. |
|---|---|---|---|---|
| | MK2 | | | 1 |
| | GMFb | | | 1 |
| | cyclinA | | | 2 |
| | TCP | | | 2 |
| | EGF | | | 2 |
| | H4 | | | 2 |
| | actin | | | 2 |
| | GRg2 | | | 2 |
| | IGFR2 | | | 2 |
| | FABP | | | 2 |
| | GAD65 | | | 2 |
| | GRg3 | | | 2 |
| | InsR | | | 2 |
| | ODC | | | 2 |
| | IGF2 | | | 2 |
| | CCO2 | | | 2 |
| | CNTF | | | 2 |
| | CNTFR | | | 2 |
| | CX43 | | | 3 |
| | bFGF | | Krox-24 | 3 |
| | GRa2 | | | 3 |
| | IP3R2 | | | 3 |
| | synaptophysin | | | 3 |
| | ACHE | | Krox-24 | 3 |
| | neno | | Krox-24 | 3 |
| | IGF1 | | | 3 |
| | GAD67 | | Krox-24 | 3 |
| | preGAD67 | | | 3 |
| | 5HT1b | | | 3 |
| | NT3 | | | 3 |
| | mGluR3 | | | 3 |
| | nAChRa5 | | | 3 |
| | GRa4 | | | 3 |
| | nAChRa7 | | Krox-24 | 3 |
| | GRg1 | | | 3 |
| | cjun | | | 4 |
| | CCO1 | | | 5 |
| | GAP43 | | | 6 |
| | GRa3 | | | 7 |
| | 5HT2 | | | 8 |
| | GRb2 | | | 8 |
| | cellubrevin | | | 9 |
| | GRa1 | | | 10 |
| | GRa5 | | | 10 |
| | GRb1 | | | 10 |
| | mAChR2 | | | 10 |
| | NFM | | | 10 |
| | NFH | | | 10 |
| | NFL | | Krox-24 | 10 |
| | S100beta | | | 10 |
| | GFAP | | | 10 |
| | mGluR8 | | | 11 |
| | cyclinB | | | 12 |
| | nestin | | | 12 |
| | G67I8086 | | | 12 |
| | G67I86 | | | 12 |
| | Brm | | | 12 |
| | TH | | | 12 |
| | IGFR1 | | | 12 |
| | nAChRa3 | | | 12 |
| | IP3R3 | | | 13 |
| | 5HT3 | | | 13 |
| | trkC | | | 14 |
| | mAChR1 | | | 14 |
| | GRb3 | | | 14 |
| | PDGFb | | | 15 |
| | PDGFR | | | 15 |
| | aFGF | | | 15 |
| | BDNF | | | 16 |
| | MOG | | | 16 |

**Figure 11.4** Three alternative methods for the clustering of developmental hippocampus gene expression data. (*A*) Gene expression patterns were normalized to their respective minima and maxima, and clustered using an agglomerative algorithm. (*B*) Gene expression patterns were normalized to their respective maxima and clustered using

**C**

| Gene | E15 | E18 | P0 | P3 | P7 | P10 | P13 | P25 | A | Cis-element | Cluster no. |
|---|---|---|---|---|---|---|---|---|---|---|---|
| MOG | | | | | | | | | | | 1 |
| 5HT3 | | | | | | | | | | | 2 |
| aFGF | | | | | | | | | | | 2 |
| GRb3 | | | | | | | | | | | 2 |
| IP3R3 | | | | | | | | | | | 2 |
| PDGFb | | | | | | | | | | | 2 |
| PDGFR | | | | | | | | | | | 2 |
| mAChR1 | | | | | | | | | | | 3 |
| nAChRa3 | | | | | | | | | | | 3 |
| trkC | | | | | | | | | | | 3 |
| BDNF | | | | | | | | | | | 4 |
| Brm | | | | | | | | | | | 5 |
| cyclinB | | | | | | | | | | | 5 |
| G67I8086 | | | | | | | | | | | 5 |
| G67I86 | | | | | | | | | | | 5 |
| IGFR1 | | | | | | | | | | | 5 |
| nestin | | | | | | | | | | | 5 |
| TH | | | | | | | | | | | 5 |
| ACHE | | | | | | | | | | Krox-24 | 6 |
| actin | | | | | | | | | | | 6 |
| CCO1 | | | | | | | | | | | 6 |
| CCO2 | | | | | | | | | | | 6 |
| cellubrevin | | | | | | | | | | | 6 |
| cjun | | | | | | | | | | | 6 |
| CNTF | | | | | | | | | | | 6 |
| CNTFR | | | | | | | | | | | 6 |
| CX43 | | | | | | | | | | | 6 |
| cyclinA | | | | | | | | | | | 6 |
| EGF | | | | | | | | | | | 6 |
| FABP | | | | | | | | | | | 6 |
| GAD65 | | | | | | | | | | | 6 |
| GAP43 | | | | | | | | | | | 6 |
| GMFb | | | | | | | | | | | 6 |
| GRa3 | | | | | | | | | | | 6 |
| GRg2 | | | | | | | | | | | 6 |
| GRg3 | | | | | | | | | | | 6 |
| H4 | | | | | | | | | | | 6 |
| IGF1 | | | | | | | | | | | 6 |
| IGF2 | | | | | | | | | | | 6 |
| IGFR2 | | | | | | | | | | | 6 |
| InsR | | | | | | | | | | | 6 |
| MK2 | | | | | | | | | | | 6 |
| neno | | | | | | | | | | Krox-24 | 6 |
| ODC | | | | | | | | | | | 6 |
| synaptophysin | | | | | | | | | | | 6 |
| TCP | | | | | | | | | | | 6 |
| GFAP | | | | | | | | | | | 7 |
| mGluR8 | | | | | | | | | | | 7 |
| NFH | | | | | | | | | | | 7 |
| NFL | | | | | | | | | | Krox-24 | 7 |
| S100beta | | | | | | | | | | | 7 |
| 5HT1b | | | | | | | | | | | 8 |
| 5HT2 | | | | | | | | | | | 8 |
| bFGF | | | | | | | | | | Krox-24 | 8 |
| GAD67 | | | | | | | | | | Krox-24 | 8 |
| GRa1 | | | | | | | | | | | 8 |
| GRa2 | | | | | | | | | | | 8 |
| GRa4 | | | | | | | | | | | 8 |
| GRa5 | | | | | | | | | | | 8 |
| GRb1 | | | | | | | | | | | 8 |
| GRb2 | | | | | | | | | | | 8 |
| GRg1 | | | | | | | | | | | 8 |
| IP3R2 | | | | | | | | | | | 8 |
| mAChR2 | | | | | | | | | | | 8 |
| mGluR3 | | | | | | | | | | | 8 |
| nAChRa5 | | | | | | | | | | | 8 |
| nAChRa7 | | | | | | | | | | Krox-24 | 8 |
| NFM | | | | | | | | | | | 8 |
| NT3 | | | | | | | | | | | 8 |
| preGAD67 | | | | | | | | | | | 8 |

an agglomerative algorithm. (*C*) Gene expression patterns were normalized to their respective maxima and clustered using a numerical k-means algorithm. Note the position of the genes sharing a Krox-24 transcriptional regulatory element within the clusters.

clustering, the user must define the cluster depth. Another method, k-means clustering, is optimized to identify the cluster boundaries once the number of clusters has been defined (k-means is described in standard multivariate analysis references). We used k-means clustering for figure 11.4C.

One way by which the quality of the clustering can be assessed is to compare the groupings with another indicator of gene similarity. For example, 6 genes out of the 70 are known to be regulated by the krox-24 transcriptional regulatory element. Note that these 6 genes are found within one cluster in figure 11.4A, are distributed across two clusters in figure 11.4B (one cluster containing 5 out of the 6), and are spread over three clusters in figure 11.4C. One may conclude that whereas the clustering in figure 11.4C may provide the most visually satisfying arrangement of similar patterns, the analysis in figure 11.4A provides a better description of gene similarity, as confirmed through shared control elements.

Another parameter that helps to assess cluster quality is functional gene classification. One may conjecture that genes that share common functions should be regulated together. Indeed, when examining figure 11.5, we see that certain functional gene families dominate expression clusters (highlighted by boxes). For example, the neurotransmitter receptors make up the relative majority of genes in clusters 2, 3, and 8 of the clustering methods shown in figure 11.4. Overall, the relationship between function and expression cluster mapping seems to be most optimized across all classes for the last group of k-means clustered genes.

The methods of normalization and clustering outlined here provide us with different though related results. While one method may perform ideally with respect to one criterion of cluster quality, another method may perform better according to other criteria. In other words, there may not be one globally "correct" or "optimal" method for conducting this analysis. The analysis is perhaps best carried out empirically using a variety of methods, giving us the opportunity to learn from each.

| cluster no. | neuroglial markers | transmitter receptors | peptide signaling | diverse |
|---|---|---|---|---|
| **minmaxnorm agglomerative** | | | | |
| 1 | 30% | 19% | 24% | **58%** |
| 2 | 55% | **76%** | 29% | 17% |
| 3 | | | 6% | |
| 4 | 5% | | | |
| 5 | | | | 8% |
| 6 | 5% | | 6% | 8% |
| 7 | 5% | | **24%** | 8% |
| 8 | | 5% | 12% | |
| **maxnorm agglomerative** | | | | |
| 1 | | | 12% | |
| 2 | 15% | 10% | 35% | **42%** |
| 3 | 25% | **33%** | 18% | 17% |
| 4 | | | | 8% |
| 5 | | | | 8% |
| 6 | 5% | | | |
| 7 | | 5% | | |
| 8 | | 10% | | |
| 9 | 5% | | | |
| 10 | **25%** | 19% | | |
| 11 | | 5% | | |
| 12 | **20%** | 5% | 6% | 17% |
| 13 | | 5% | | 8% |
| 14 | | **10%** | 6% | |
| 15 | | | 18% | |
| 16 | 5% | | 6% | |
| **maxnorm k–means** | | | | |
| 1 | 5% | | | |
| 2 | | 10% | **18%** | 8% |
| 3 | | 10% | 6% | |
| 4 | | | 6% | |
| 5 | **20%** | | 6% | 17% |
| 6 | 40% | 14% | 53% | **67%** |
| 7 | **20%** | 5% | | |
| 8 | 15% | **62%** | 12% | 8% |

**Figure 11.5** Functional pathways associate with coexpression clusters. The genes analyzed in figure 11.4 can be categorized according to four functional categories (column labels). The table shows the distribution of each functional category across the coexpression clusters according to the clustering methods shown in figure 11.4. The dominant functional categories for each expression cluster are highlighted with boxes.

### Reverse Engineering of Genetic Regulatory Networks from Expression Data

Ultimately, we seek to go beyond classification schemes in our analysis and find methods that predict molecular interactions. How much, and what sort of data are needed in order to unravel the regulatory interactions between genes? To a large extent, the answer will depend on the sort of analysis used. Table 11.1 lists asymptotic growth rates for clustering (represented by a correlation-based method), compared with gene network inference using various network models. The amount of data needed for clustering scales as the log of the number of genes. For network inference, it is clear that restricting the connectivity of the network model is crucial, resulting again in a logarithmic scaling with the number of genes and linear scaling with the connectivity.

It is important to keep in mind that these estimates hold for independently chosen data points and only indicate asymptotic growth rates; they ignore any constant factor. In practice, the amount of data may need to be orders of magnitude higher because of nonindependence and large measurement errors.

To correctly infer the regulation of a single gene, we need to observe the expression of that gene under many different combinations of expression levels of its regulatory inputs. Similarly, gene network inference requires a wide variety of different environmental conditions and perturbations. Measurement of gene expression time series has the valuable feature of yielding large amounts of data. However, all the data points in a single time series tend to be for a single dynamic process and will be related to the surrounding time points. A dataset of ten expression measurements under different environmental conditions, or with different mutations, will actually contain more information than a time series of ten data points on a single phenomenon.

Whereas time series data can provide crucial insights into the dynamics of the process and may allow us more easily to derive causal relationships among genes, steady-state data points may allow a more efficient mapping of the global state space. Both

**Table 11.1** Scaling of data requirements with respect to the number of genes ($N$) and estimated number of regulatory inputs per gene ($K$) in a genetic regulatory network

| MODEL | DATA NEEDED (LOWER BOUNDS) | DATA ESTIMATED FOR $N = 100$ GENES | DATA ESTIMATED FOR $N = 1000$ GENES | DATA ESTIMATED FOR $N = 10,000$ GENES | REFERENCES |
|---|---|---|---|---|---|
| Pairwise correlation (clustering) | $\log(N)$ | 6–10 | 7–12 | 8–14 | D'haeseleer, 1999a; D'haeseleer et al., 2000 |
| Boolean, fully connected | $2^N$ | $10^{30}$ | $10^{301}$ | $10^{3010}$ | |
| Boolean, connectivity $K$ | $2^K \times [K + \log(N)]$ | 165–737 | 197–865 | 229–993 | D'haeseleer, 1999a; D'haeseleer, et al., 2000; Liang et al., 1998; Akutsu et al., 1999 |
| Boolean, linearly separable, connectivity $K$ | $K \times \log(N/K)$ | 29–37 | 45–60 | 62–84 | Hertz, 1998 |
| Continuous, additive, fully connected | $N + 1$ | 101 | 1001 | 10,001 | |
| Continuous, additive, connectivity $K$ | $K \times \log(N/K)$? | 29–37 | 45–60 | 62–84 | D'haeseleer, 1999a; D'haeseleer et al., 2000 |

*Notes:* These growth rates are lower bounds, valid for large $N$, and ignoring any constant factors. The concrete values in the last three columns are for illustration purposes only, calculated from the more precise formulas in D'haeseleer et al. (2000) and Hertz (1998) using $K = 5$ to 7 and a few other commonsense assumptions. Pairwise correlation: assign genes to the same cluster if their correlation exceeds a given threshold (stand-in for clustering in general); Boolean: Boolean network; Continuous: continuous-valued (e.g., differential equation) model; Linearly separable, additive: gene regulation modeled by weighted sum of inputs (simple thresholding behavior).

types of data, and multiple data sets of each, will likely be needed to decipher the regulatory networks.

Fitting a single model of the gene network to several datasets from the same organism raises another set of problems. Most current datasets contain relative expression levels—relative to a different reference mRNA population for each dataset. Clearly, if we want to compare or combine datasets, there is an urgent need for the development of a common reference. In addition, strains and environmental conditions should be as standardized and controlled as possible to allow changes in environmental variables to be incorporated into the model.

As an example of how gene network inference can be applied to real data, we have constructed a very simple, linear model of a relatively small number of genes in the rat CNS, fitted to three separate time series: development of rat cervical spinal cord (112 genes, 9 data points from embryonic day 11 through adult) (Wen et al., 1998); development of rat hippocampus (70 genes, 9 data points from embryonic day 15 through adult); and kainate injury in rat hippocampus (70 genes, 10 data points from injection at postnatal day 25 to 49 days after injection) (Fuhrman et al., 2000).

We modeled the change in gene expression at each time step as a weighted sum of expression levels at the previous time step:

$$\frac{X_i(t + \Delta t) - X_i(t)}{\Delta t} = \sum_j W_{ji} X_j(t) + K_i \times \text{kainate}(t) + T_i \times \text{tissue} + C_i$$

where $X_i(t)$ is the expression level of gene $i$ at time $t$. Parameter $W_{ji}$ accounts for the influence of the expression level of gene $j$ on the expression level of gene $i$. The variable kainate($t$) models the kainate level during the kainate injury experiment. Parameter $K_i$ models the effect of the presence of kainate-induced seizure on gene $i$. The variable tissue is 0 for the spinal cord time series and 1 for the hippocampus time series. Parameter $T_i$ accounts for the differences in expression of gene $i$ that are due to tissue type, and parameter $C_i$ is a bias constant indicating the expression level of gene $i$ in the absence of any other regulatory inputs.

We interpolated the nonequidistant data points in the three time series up to a very fine time step $\Delta t$ (6 minutes) and then fit the parameters in the model to the interpolated data using a least-squares approximation.

The results obtained using this simple linear fitting have some very plausible general properties: (1) The weight matrix $W$ is sparse, that is, most interaction weights are close to 0 (each gene is affected by only a small number of regulatory inputs). (2) Most genes have both positive and negative regulatory inputs. (3) Some genes are biased toward a predominantly positive or predominantly negative regulatory effect. (4) Some of the main regulatory gene categories are neurotransmitter metabolizing enzymes and glutamate receptors. (5) Genes in a functional class tend to receive more inputs from genes in the same class.

We also found that it is possible to initialize the model with the very first gene expression levels measured in each of the time series and to reconstruct the original trajectories by applying the model iteratively (figure 11.6). Furthermore, the model will converge to the correct adult expression levels, which can be verified by analyzing the eigenvectors of the system (see D'haeseleer et al., 1999, for a more in-depth analysis of these results).

Of course, it might seem that fitting a 65-variable model using only 28 data points would lead to a grossly underconstrained system. The situation is not quite as bad as it seems, however, because the (cubic) interpolation used in effect imposes an extra smoothness constraint on the time series in between the actual measurements. Given this additional constraint, there is only a single optimal solution for the parameters.

We still expect large parts of the model to be poorly constrained, so we used a perturbation analysis to determine the most robust parameters. The original data consists of triplicate experiments, which gives us a rough estimate of the standard deviation on each measurement. We constructed 40 new input datasets, with a small amount of Gaussian noise added to each measurement, and generated the linear model for each of these perturbed datasets. This

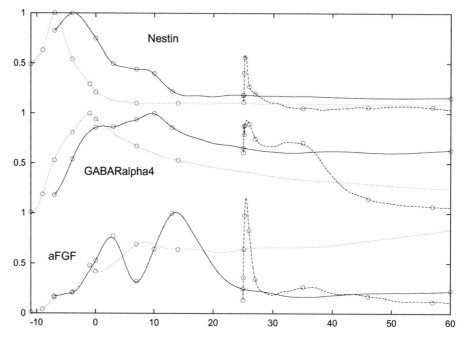

**Figure 11.6** Time series reconstructed by the model for three different genes. Hollow circles are original data points. Dotted, reconstruction of cervical spinal cord development (time in days, birth = 0); solid, hippocampus development; dashed, hippocampus kainate injury.

allowed us to analyze the noise sensitivity of each parameter in the input data.

Surprisingly, the most robust parameters (smallest coefficient of variation over the 40 perturbed models) are the ones accounting for the effect of kainate on each gene (parameters $K_i$). This is probably because of the very fast and drastic effect of kainate-induced seizures on the system, compared with the slow and subtle changes during development. The six kainate parameters with the highest robustness and absolute value are summarized in table 11.2, and are discussed in the following paragraphs (a more detailed analysis of these results is in preparation [D'haeseleer and Fuhrman, unpublished data]).

**Table 11.2** Six kainate parameters with high robustness and high absolute value

| PARAMETER | VALUE |
|---|---|
| Kainate $\rightarrow$ IGF II | $-1.16$ |
| Kainate $\rightarrow$ BDNF | $+0.75$ |
| Kainate $\rightarrow$ TCP | $+0.54$ |
| Kainate $\rightarrow$ S100$\beta$ | $+0.53$ |
| Kainate $\rightarrow$ G67I86 | $+0.38$ |
| Kainate $\rightarrow$ 5-HT$_{1B}$ | $+0.21$ |

*Notes:* Positive value indicates upregulation by kainate. Negative value indicates downregulation. TCP, T-complex protein.

## Kainate $\longrightarrow$ IGF II

Kar and colleagues (1997) suggested a possible involvement of insulin, insulin-like growth factor (IGF) I, and IGF II in the cascade of neurotrophic events that is associated with the reorganization of the hippocampal formation observed following kainate-induced seizures. We found a fourfold decrease in IGF II mRNA levels after one-half hour, followed by a large decrease of all IGFs and IGF receptors after about 10 to 21 days. Clearly, IGF II should be considered an immediate early gene, and its significant underexpression may be involved in the downregulation of the IGF receptors over time.

## Kainate $\longrightarrow$ BDNF

Brain-derived neurotrophic factor (BDNF) is known to be upregulated as an immediate early gene by kainate (Nakayama et al., 1994; Castren et al., 1998), and is thought to play a major role in kainate-induced damage to the hippocampus in the adult brain. Administration of antisense BDNF after kainate administration prevents neuronal hypertrophy (Guilhem et al., 1996), and hippocampal BDNF levels are correlated with the severity of seizures and neuronal loss in CA1 and CA3 (Rudge et al., 1998).

### Kainate —→ TCP

Little evidence can be found in the literature for kainate regulation of T-complex protein (TCP). One intriguing link is the mapping of the epilepsy susceptibility locus EJM1 on chromosome 6 (Sander et al., 1997), near a human homologue of the mouse T-complex (Durner et al., 1992). If TCP indeed plays a role in kainate-induced seizures, TCP gene defects might also cause increased susceptibility to epilepsy.

### Kainate —→ S100$\beta$

S100$\beta$ is upregulated fivefold in human temporal lobe epilepsy (Griffin et al., 1995) and is known to protect hippocampal neurons from damage induced by glucose deprivation (Barger et al., 1995), so its overexpression may be a consequence of glucose deprivation that is due to neuronal hyperexcitation by kainate. S100$\beta$ overexpression may also aggravate the effects of kainate because it induces apoptotic cell death in astrocytes (Hu and Van Eldik, 1996), which protect against kainate neurotoxicity (Mattson and Rychlik, 1990).

### Kainate —→ G67I86

G67I86 is an embryonic splice variant of GAD67 (Bond et al., 1990). Mature GAD67 mRNA is known to be upregulated in hippocampal dentate granule cells 4 hours after kainate injection (Schwartzer and Sperk, 1995; Ding et al., 1998). We found that G67I86 mRNA levels increase first, followed by a second embryonic splice variant, and finally the adult mRNA, which is exactly the same sequence in which these variants appear during development (Szabo et al., 1994). Recapitulations of developmental processes play an important role in regeneration of the peripheral nervous system and have also been implicated in the central nervous system (Cohen and Hall, 1986; Yang et al., 1997).

### Kainate $\longrightarrow$ 5-HT$_{1B}$

Kainate administration causes serotonin release in the hippocampus (Tao et al., 1997). Activation of the 5-HT$_{1B}$ autoreceptor results in (1) inhibition of serotonin release (Johanning et al., 1992), (2) desensitization of the 5-HT$_{1B}$ receptor (Pleus and Bylund, 1992), and possibly (3) an additional compensatory downregulation of the receptor (Johanning et al., 1992). This complex set of regulatory feedback loops (each presumably operating on different time scales) may very well cause an initial upregulation of 5-HT$_{1B}$ mRNA levels. Indeed, the 5-HT$_{1B}$ time series shows a transient upregulation, followed by the expected decrease below the initial expression level.

The gene-to-gene interactions (parameters $W_{ji}$) predicted by the model are typically much less robust than the kainate parameters (greater coefficient of variation over the 40 perturbed models). Furthermore, whereas the effects of kainate are well studied, typically less is known about the regulatory relationships between any two genes, so the evidence for these interactions in the existing literature is much less clear. The ten most robust gene-to-gene interactions are summarized in table 11.3. Some of the results are quite intriguing, such as apparent autoregulation of two genes (GFAP and BDNF); mutually inhibitory regulation among three genes that may be involved in differentiation into different neuronal cell types (BDNF, IGF II, and S100$\beta$); and apparent coordinate regulation of a possible $\alpha4\beta2\gamma1$ GABA-A receptor, two neurotransmitter metabolizing enzymes (acetylcholinesterase and embryonic glutamic acid decarboxylase 67 splice variants), and a neuronal marker, neurofilament medium (NFM) by the $\gamma1$ GABA-A receptor subtype. A more detailed analysis of these results is in preparation (D'haeseleer and Fuhrman, unpublished data).

**Table 11.3** Most robust gene-to-gene interactions

| PARAMETER | VALUE |
| --- | --- |
| GFAP → GFAP | −0.28 |
| BDNF, IGF II → BDNF, S100β | Negative |
| GRγ1 → GRα4, GRβ2, G67I80/86, AChE, NFM | Positive |

**Conclusion**

This chapter has examined several levels of analysis of gene expression data, each with unique applications to the discovery of important molecular processes. Beginning with simple differential expression studies covering only a handful of conditions, one may seek to simply identify the genes that show significant fluctuations of expression.

A more complex fluctuation analysis can be carried out for larger datasets using the Shannon entropy measure. Using this method, genes may be identified that allow us to optimally distinguish physiological processes, tissues, and various treatments. Many of these genes are likely to be important physiological players in these processes.

On the opposite end of the scale, we may seek to group the genes most similar in their expression patterns to capture functional pathways and reduce the complexity of the expression data. Often we find that genes with similar expression profiles originate from the same or related gene families. Through coexpression clustering we strive to infer connections between pathways and identify new pathways that link genes that were previously thought to be unrelated.

Ultimately, we seek to directly infer important regulatory relationships between genes from activity profiles. We have examined a straightforward linear modeling method that has resulted in several plausible predictions of gene interaction, some of which can be verified through comparison with the existing experimental literature.

There are several challenges that we must still face in determining the data requirements and appropriate experimental design for our analytical approaches. These new measurement and analysis technologies require new experimental design approaches to gain maximal insight. Ideally, every set of predictions from an analysis should be the basis for future experimental designs. These will lead to the extension or revision of models, resulting, it is hoped, in significant improvements—to the point where our models become truly predictive and reliable.

## References

Akutsu T, Miyano S, and Kuhara S (1999). Identification of genetic networks from a small number of gene expression pattern under the Boolean network model. Presented at Pacific Symposium on Biocomputing, Kohala Coast, Hawaii, January 1999. *Proceedings, Pacific Symposium on Biocomputing*. Altman RB, Lauderdale K, Dunker AK, Hunter L, Klein TE, eds. World Scientific Publishing Co. Pte. Ltd., Singapore, pp 17–28. (available at http://www.smi.stanford.edu/projects/helix/psb99/Akutsu.pdf)

Barger SW, Van Eldik LJ, and Mattson MP (1995). S100 beta protects hippocampal neurons against damage induced by glucose deprivation. *Brain Res* 667: 167–70.

Bond RW, Wyborski RJ, and Gottlieb DI (1990). Developmentally regulated expression of an exon containing a stop codon in the gene for glutamic acid decarboxylase. *Proc Nat Acad Sci USA* 87: 8771–75.

Castren E, Berninger B, Leingartner A, and Lindholm D (1998). Regulation of brain-derived neurotrophic factor mRNA levels in hippocampus by neuronal activity. *Prog Brain Res* 117: 57–64.

Cohen MJ and Hall GF (1986). Control of neuron shape during development and regeneration. *Neurochem Pathol* 5: 331–43.

D'haeseleer P (1999a). Data requirements for inferring genetic networks from expression data. Presented at Pacific Symposium on Biocomputing, Kohala Coast, Hawaii, January 1999. (available at http://www.cs.unm.edu/~patrik/networks/PSB99/poster.html)

D'haeseleer P, Wen X, Fuhrman S, and Somogyi R (1999b). Linear modeling of mRNA expression levels during CNS development and injury. Presented at Pacific Symposium on Biocomputing, Kohala Coast, Hawaii, January 1999. *Proceedings, Pacific Symposium on Biocomputing*. World Scientific Publishing Co. Pte. Ltd., Singapore, pp 41–52.

D'haeseleer P, Liang S, and Somogyi R (2000). Genetic network inference: from co-expression clustering to reverse engineering. *Bioinformatics* 16: 707–26.

Ding R, Asada H, and Obata K (1998). Changes in extracellular glutamate and GABA levels in the hippocampal CA3 and CA1 areas and the induction of glutamic acid decarboxylase-67 in dentate granule cells of rats treated with kainic acid. *Brain Res* 800: 105–13.

Durner M, Greenberg DA, and Delgado-Escueta AV (1992). Is there a genetic relationship between epilepsy and birth defects? *Neurology* 42(4 suppl 5): 63–67.

Fuhrman S, Cunningham MJ, Wen X, Zweiger G, Seilhamer JJ, and Somogyi R (2000). The application of Shannon entropy in the identification of putative drug targets. *Biosystems* 55: 5–14.

Griffin WS, Yeralan O, Sheng JG, Boop FA, Mrak RE, Rovnaghi CR, et al. (1995). Overexpression of the neurotrophic cytokine S100 beta in human temporal lobe epilepsy. *J Neurochem* 65: 228–33.

Guilhem D, Dreyfus PA, Makiura Y, Suzuki F, Onteniente B (1996). Short increase of BDNF messenger RNA triggers kainic acid-induced neuronal hypertrophy in adult mice. *Neuroscience* 72: 923–31.

Hertz J (1998). Statistical issues in reverse engineering of genetic networks. Presented at Pacific Symposium on Biocomputing, Kapalua, Hawaii, January 1998. (available for downloading at: http://www.nordita.dk/~hertz/projects.html).

Hu J and Van Eldik LJ (1996). S100 beta induces apoptotic cell death in cultured astrocytes via a nitric oxide-dependent pathway. *Biochim Biophys Acta* 1313: 239–45.

Johanning H, Plenge P, Mellerup E (1992). Serotonin receptors in the brain of rats treated chronically with imipramine or RU24969: support for the 5-HT1B receptor being a 5-HT autoreceptor. *Pharmacol Toxicol* 70: 131–4.

Kar S, Seto D, Doré S, Chabot J-G, and Quirion R (1997). Systemic administration of kainic acid induces selective time-dependent decrease in [125I]insulin receptor binding sites in adult rat hippocampal formation. *Neuroscience* 80: 1041–55.

Kauffman SA (1993). *The Origins of Order*, Oxford University Press, New York.

Liang S, Fuhrman S, and Somogyi R (1998). REVEAL, A general reverse engineering algorithm for inference of genetic network architectures. Presented at Pacific Symposium on Biocomputing, Kapalua, Hawaii, January 1998. *Proceedings, Pacific Symposium on Biocomputing*. Altman RB, Dunker AK, Hunter L, Klein TE, eds. World Scientific Publishing Co. Pte. Ltd., Singapore, pp 18–29.

Mattson MP and Rychlik B (1990). Glia protect hippocampal neurons against excitatory amino acid-induced degeneration: involvement of fibroblast growth factor. *Int J Dev Neurosci* 8: 399–415.

Nakayama M, Gahara Y, Kitamura T, and Ohara O (1994). Distinctive four promoters collectively direct expression of brain-derived neurotrophic factor gene. *Brain Res Mol Brain Res* 21: 206–18.

Pleus RC and Bylund DB (1992). Desensitization and down-regulation of the 5-hydroxytryptamine1B receptor in the opossum kidney cell line. *J Pharmacol Exp Ther* 261: 271–7.

Rudge JS, Mather PE, Pasnikowski EM, Cai N, Corcoran T, and Acheson A (1998). Endogenous BDNF protein is increased in adult rat hippocampus after a kainic acid induced excitotoxic insult but exogenous BDNF is not neuroprotective. *Exp Neurol* 149: 398–410.

Sander T, Bockenkamp B, Hildmann T, Blasczyk R, Kretz R, Wienker TF, et al. (1997). Refined mapping of the epilepsy susceptibility locus EJM1 on chromosome 6. *Neurology* 49: 842–7.

Schwarzer C and Sperk G (1995). Hippocampal granule cells express glutamic acid decarboxylase-67 after limbic seizures in the rat. *Neuroscience* 69: 705–9.

Shannon CE and Weaver W (1963). *The Mathematical Theory of Communication,* Univ. of Illinois Press, Chicago, IL.

Somogyi R and Sniegoski C (1996). Modeling the complexity of genetic networks: Understanding multigenic and pleiotropic regulation. *Complexity* 1: 45–63.

Szabo G, Katarova Z, and Greenspan R (1994). Distinct protein forms are produced from alternatively spliced bicistronic glutamic acid decarboxylase mRNAs during development. *Mol Cell Biol* 14: 7535–45.

Tao R, Ma Z, and Auerbach SB (1997). Influence of AMPA/kainate receptors on extracellular 5-hydroxytryptamine in rat midbrain raphe and forebrain. *Br J Pharmacol* 121: 1707–15.

Wen X, Fuhrman S, Michaels GS, Carr DB, Smith S, Barker JL, et al. (1998) Large-scale temporal gene expression mapping of central nervous system development. *Proc Nat Acad Sci USA* 95: 334–9.

Yang HY, Lieska N, Kriho V, Wu CM, and Pappas GD (1997). A subpopulation of reactive astrocytes at the immediate site of cerebral cortical injury. *Exp Neurol* 146: 199–205.

# Appendix A   Informatics and Web Resources

Noncommercial

---

**IMAGE QUANTIFICATION SOFTWARE**

---

| Product | Institution/Person | URL |
|---|---|---|
| CrazyQuant | Leroy Hood | chroma.mbt.washington.edu/mod_www/tools/ |
| DataMachine | David Strehlow | people.bu.edu/strehlow |
| ScanAlyze | Michael Eisen | rana.lbl.gov |
| TIGR Spotfinder | John Quackenbush (TIGR) | www.tigr.org |

---

**DATA ANALYSIS SOFTWARE: DATA MINING**

---

| Product | Institution/Person | URL |
|---|---|---|
| Cluster/TreeView | Michael Eisen | rana.lbl.gov |
| DataMachine | David Strehlow | people.bu.edu/strehlow |
| GeneCluster | Whitehead Institute (MIT) | www-genome.wi.mit.edu/MPR |
| GeneX | National Center for Genome Resources | www.ncgr.org |
| J-Express | Bjarte Dysvik and Inge Jonassen. | www.ii.uib.no/~bjarted/jexpress |
| Plaid Models | Laura Lazzeroni and Art Owen | www-stat.stanford.edu/~owen/plaid/ |
| The Equalizer | Robert Stuart | http://organogenesis.ucsd.edu/ |

| | | |
|---|---|---|
| dCHIP | Wing Wong | http://biosun1.harvard.edu/complab/dchip/ |
| 2HAPI | San Diego Super Computer Center | http://array.sdsc.edu/hapi_web/ |
| Dragon Database | Jonathan Pevsner | http://pevsnerlab.kennedykrieger.org/dragon.htm#example |
| Tools for Data Analysis and Visualization | John Weinstein | http://discover.nci.nih.gov/nature.2000/ |

**DATA ANALYSIS SOFTWARE: PRIMARY STATISTICAL INFERENCE**

| Product | Institution/Person | URL |
|---|---|---|
| dChip | Wing Wong | www.biostat.harvard.edu/complab/dchip/ |
| SAM | Robert Tibshirani | www-stat.stanford.edu/~tibs/SAM/index.html |
| R package: Statistics for Microarray Analysis | Terry Speed | www.stat.berkeley.edu/users/terry/zarray/Html/ |

Commercial

**IMAGE QUANTIFICATION SOFTWARE**

| Product | Company | URL |
|---|---|---|
| Array-Pro Analyzer | Media Cybernetics | www.mediacy.com |
| ArrayVision | Imaging Research | www.imagingresearch.com |
| AtlasImage | Clontech | www.clontech.com |
| GenePix | Axon Instruments | www.axon.com |
| GLEAMS | NuTec Sciences | www.nutecsciences.com |
| ImaGene/AutoGene | BioDiscovery | www.biodiscovery.com |
| IPLab, MicroArray Suite | Scanalytics | www.scanalytics.com |
| Phoretix Array | Phoretix | www.phoretix.com |

| | | |
|---|---|---|
| QuantArray | Packard Bioscience | www.packardbioscience.com |
| Gene TAC | Genomic Solutions | www.genomicsolutions.com |
| XdotsReader | Cose | www.cose.fr |
| Microarray Suite | Affymetrix | www.affymetrix.com. |

## DATA ANALYSIS SOFTWARE: PRIMARY STATISTICAL INFERENCE

| Product | Company | URL |
|---|---|---|
| ArrayStat | Imaging Research | www.imagingresearch.com |
| MicroArray Suite | Scanalytics | www.scanalytics.com |
| Resolver | Rosetta Inpharmatics | www.rii.com |

## DATA ANALYSIS SOFTWARE: DATA MINING

| Product | Company | URL |
|---|---|---|
| Decision Site | SpotFire | www.spotfire.com |
| arraySCOUT | Lion Bioscience | www.lionbioscience.com |
| AtlasNavigator | Clontech | www.clontech.com |
| CHIPSpace | Hitachi | www.miraibio.com |
| Expressionist | GeneData | www.genedata.com |
| Eosurveyor | Eos | www.eosbiotech.com |
| GeneMaths | Applied Maths | www.applied-maths.com |
| GeneSpring | Silicon Genetics | www.sigenetics.com |
| GeneSight | BioDiscovery | www.biodiscovery.com |
| GenoMax | InforMax | www.informaxinc.com |
| GLEAMS | NuTec Sciences | www.nutecsciences.com |
| Partek Pro | Partek | www.partek.com |
| Resolver | Rosetta Inpharmatics | www.rii.com |
| Data Mining Tool | Affymetrix | www.affymetrix.com |
| NetAffx | Affymetrix | www.affymetrix.com |

# Appendix B  Company and Array-Related Web Resources

## COMMERCIAL OR NONCOMMERCIAL CLONE SETS

| Product | Company/Institution | URL |
|---|---|---|
| Molecular Biology Clones | ATCC | http://phage.atcc.org/searchengine/mb.html |
| IMAGE clone sets | IMAGE Consortium | http://image.llnl.gov/ |
| IMAGE, LifeSeq, GEM clone sets | IncyteGenomics | http://www.incyte.com/reagents/catalog.jsp?page=clones/image/index |
| arrayTAG—Optimized cDNA-Probes | LION Bioscience | http://www.lionbioscience.com/htm/c_1/index_c_1.htm |
| NIA Mouse 15K cDNA clone set | NIA | http://lgsun.grc.nia.nih.gov/cDNA/15k.html |
| I.M.A.G.E. Consortium cDNA Clones | Research Genetics (Invitrogen) | http://www.resgen.com |
| Human Neuroarray (6K set) | | http://www.resgen.com http://geschwindlab.medsch.ucla.edu |
| Mouse Full-length cDNA clones | Riken | http://genome.rtc.riken.go.jp. |

## PREFORMATTED ARRAYS

| Product | Company/Institution | URL |
|---|---|---|
| GeneChip Arrays | Affymetrix | http://www.affymetrix.com/products/app_exp.html |
| Microarrays (oligonucleotide, cDNA) | Agilent Technologies | http://www.chem.agilent.com/Scripts/Generic.ASP?lPage=416 |
| Human ULTRArray Membrane | Ambion, Inc. | http://www.ambion.com/catalog/CatNum.php?3150 |

| | | |
|---|---|---|
| Atlas Arrays | Clontech, Inc. | http://www.clontech.com/atlas/atlasglass/index.html |
| GeneMap Preprinted Microarrays | Genomic Solutions, Inc. | http://www.genomicsolutions.com/products/bio/genemap.html |
| NIEHS Chips | NIEHS | http://dir.niehs.nih.gov/microarray/chips.htm |
| OpArrays | Operon Technologies, Inc. | http://www.operon.com/arrays/arraystock.php |
| Micromax cDNA Microarrays | Perkin Elmer Life Sciences (NEN Life Sciences) | http://www.nen.com/products/micromax/micro_index.htm |
| Phase-1 Microarrays | Phase-1 Molecular Toxicology, Inc. | http://www.phase1tox.com/products.html |
| Protogene Microarrays | Protogene Laboratories, Inc. | http://www.protogene.com/products/index.shtml |
| DNA Expression Arrays | R&D Systems, Inc. | http://www.rndsystems.com/asp/c_search.asp |
| Mammalian GeneFilters Microarrays | Research Genetics | http://www.resgen.com/products/MammGF.php3 |
| FlexJet DNA Microarrays | Rosetta Inpharmatics | http://www.rii.com/prodserv/inkjet/default.htm |
| Arrays | Spectral Genomics, Inc. | http://www.spectralgenomics.com/ |

## ARRAYERS

| *Product* | *Company* | *URL* |
|---|---|---|
| Generation III Array Spotter | AP Biotech (Molecular Dynamics, Inc.) | http://www.apbiotech.com/application/microarray/ |
| MicroGrid, BioGrid | BioRobotics | http://www.biorobotics.co.uk/ |
| Cartesian Microarray Spotting Workstation | Cartesian Technologies | http://www.cartesiantech.com/microarray_products.htm |
| OmniGrid | GeneMachines | http://www.genemachines.com/OmniGrid/OmniGrid.html |
| Q Bot, Q Pix, Q Array | Genetix | http://www.genetix.co.uk/Instruments.htm |
| GeneTAC G$^3$ Robotic Workstation | Genomic Solutions, Inc. | http://www.genomicsolutions.com/products/bio/g3.html |

| High Throughput Micro Arraying | Intelligent Automation Systems | http://www.intelligentbio.com/ |
| BioChip Arrayer | Packard Instrument Company | http://www.packardbiochip.com/products/biochip_arrayer.htm |
| SpotBot Microarrayer | TeleChem International, Inc. | http://www.arrayit.com/Chem_Array/Arrayit_Brand_Products/Spotting_Products/SpotBot/spotbot.html |
| ChipWriter | Virtek Vision International, Inc. | http://www.virtekvision.com/ |

## SCANNERS

| *Product* | *Company* | *URL* |
| --- | --- | --- |
| DNA Microarray Scanner | Agilent Technologies | http://www.chem.agilent.com/Scripts/PDS.asp?IPage=398 |
| FluorChem, AlphaArray | Alpha Innotech Corporation | http://www.alphainnotech.com/bio/lsmaster.html |
| Array Scanner | AP Biotech (Molecular Dynamics, Inc.) | http://www.apbiotech.com/application/microarray/ |
| ArrayWoRx Microarray Scanner | Applied Precision, Inc. | http://www.api.com/dvarrayworx.html |
| GenePix Array Scanner | Axon Instruments, Inc. | http://www.axon.com/GN_Genomics.html#scanner |
| DNAscope | GeneFocus | http://www.genefocus.com/products_and_specifications.htm |
| GeneTAC Biochip Analyzer | Genomic Solutions, Inc. | http://www.genomicsolutions.com/products/bio/img.html |
| ScanArray | Packard Instrument Company | http://www.packardbiochip.com/products/products.htm |
| ChipReader | Virtek Vision International, Inc. | http://www.virtekvision.com/ |

## AUTOMATED HYBRIDIZATION STATIONS

| Product | Company | URL |
|---|---|---|
| Automated Slide Processor | AP Biotech (Molecular Dynamics, Inc.) | http://www.apbiotech.com/ application/microarray/ |
| GeneTAC Hybridization Station | Genomic Solutions, Inc. | http://www.genomicsolutions.com/ products/bio/hyb.html |

## SPECIALTY SUPPLIES AND REAGENTS

| Product | Company | URL |
|---|---|---|
| RNA prep reagents | Ambion, Inc. | http://www.ambion.com/ |
| Slides, hybridization supplies, labeling reagents | AP Biotech (Molecular Dynamics, Inc.) | http://www.apbiotech.com/ application/microarray/ |
| Slides, hybridization supplies | Corning, Inc. | http://www.corning.com/CMT/ |
| 3DNA signal amplification | Genisphere, Inc. | http://www.genisphere.com/ ExpressionArrays.html |
| Hybridization supplies, membrane-coated slides | Grace BioLabs | http://www.gracebio.com/ products.html |
| RNA prep reagents | Invitrogen | http://www.invitrogen.com/ catalog_project/index.html |
| RNA prep reagents, SuperScript II reverse transcriptase | Life Technologies, Inc. (Gibco BRL) | http://www.lifetech.com |
| Fluorescent nucleotides | Molecular Probes | http://www.molecularprobes.com/ |
| General array technology | Oxford Gene Technology | http://www.ogt.co.uk/home.html |
| TSA labeling kit, fluorescent nucleotides, slides | Perkin Elmer Life Sciences (NEN Life Sciences) | http://www.nen.com/products/ micromax/prod_serv.htm |
| RNA prep reagents, reverse transcription reagents, DNA prep reagents, dye removal kit | Qiagen, Inc. | http://www.qiagen.com/array/ index.html |
| Membrane-coated slides | Schleicher & Schuell | http://www.s-und-s.de/Pages-NEU-eng/UB3/Life%20Science/ micarray.htm |
| Arrayer pins, slides, hybridization supplies, DNA prep reagents | TeleChem International, Inc. | http://www.arrayit.com/ |

## ACADEMIC RESOURCES AND LINK SITES

| Site | URL |
| --- | --- |
| Brown Lab | http://cmgm.stanford.edu/pbrown/ |
| European Bioinformatics Institute | http://www.ebi.ac.uk/ |
| Gene Expression Omnibus | http://www.ncbi.nlm.nih.gov/geo/ |
| Grid It Resources for Microarray Technology | http://www.bsi.vt.edu/ralscher/gridit/ |
| Leming Shi's DNA Microarray Page | http://www.gene-chips.com/ |
| Microarray (Y. F. Leung's Functional Genomics Site) | http://ihome.cuhk.edu.ht/~b400559/ |
| Microarrays.org | http://microarrays.org/index.html |
| National Institute of Environmental Health Science | http://dir.niehs.nih.gov/microarray/ |
| National Center for Genome Resources | http://www.ncgr.org/research/genex/other_tools.html |
| NHGRI Microarray Project | http://www.nhgri.nih.gov/DIR/LCG/15K/HTML/ |
| The Institute for Genome Research (TIGR) | http://www.tigr.org/tdb/microarray/ |
| Stanford Microarray Database | http://genome-www4.stanford.edu/MicroArray/SMD/ |
| Vanderbilt University | http://array.mc.vanderbilt.edu/ |

# Contributors

**Tarif A. Awad**  Affymetrix, Inc., Santa Clara, California

**Carrolee Barlow**  Laboratory of Genetics, The Salk Institute for Biological Studies, La Jolla, California

**Tanya Barrett**  Transgenic Knockout Facility, National Institute on Aging, National Institutes of Health, Baltimore, Maryland

**Trent Basarsky**  Axon Instruments, Inc., Union City, California

**Kevin G. Becker**  DNA Array Unit, National Institute on Aging, National Institutes of Health, Baltimore, Maryland

**Bruno Cauli**  Neurobiologie et Diversité Cellulaire, Centre National de la Recherche Scientifique UMR7637, ESPCI, Paris, France

**Lillian W. Chiang**  Millennium Pharmaceuticals, Inc., Cambridge, Massachusetts

**Patrik D'haeseleer**  Department of Computer Science, University of New Mexico, Albuquerque, New Mexico

**Frédéric Devaux**  Laboratoire de Génétique Moléculaire, Centre National de la Recherche Scientifique UMR8541, ENS, Paris, France

**Dave Ficenec**          Millennium Pharmaceuticals, Inc., Cambridge, Massachusetts

**Stefanie Fuhrman**      Molecular Mining Corporation, Kingston, Ontario, Canada

**Daniel H. Geschwind**   Neurogenetics Program, Department of Neurology, UCLA School of Medicine, Los Angeles, California

**Nathalie Gibelin**      Neurobiologie et Diversité Cellulaire, Centre National de la Recherche Scientifique UMR7637, ESPCI, Paris, France

**Stephen D. Ginsberg**   Departments of Pediatrics and Neuroscience, Baylor College of Medicine, Houston, Texas

**Geoffroy Golfier**      Neurobiologie et Diversité Cellulaire, Centre National de la Recherche Scientifique UMR7637, ESPCI, Paris, France

**Jeffrey P. Gregg**      Department of Pathology, UC Davis School of Medicine, Sacramento, California

**Jill M. Grenier**       Millennium Pharmaceuticals, Inc., Cambridge, Massachusetts

**Hermann Hubschle**      Imaging Research, Inc., St. Catharines, Ontario, Canada

**Sonia Kuhlmann**        Neurobiologie et Diversité Cellulaire, Centre National de la Recherche Scientifique UMR7637, ESPCI, Paris, France

**Bertrand Lambolez**     Neurobiologie et Diversité Cellulaire, Centre National de la Recherche Scientifique UMR7637, ESPCI, Paris, France

| | |
|---|---|
| **Béatrice Le Bourdellès** | Neuroscience Research Centre, Merck, Sharp, & Dohme Research Laboratories, Terlings Park, Harlow, UK |
| **Virginia M.-Y. Lee** | Center for Neurodegenerative Disease Research, Department of Pathology and Laboratory Medicine, University of Pennsylvania School of Medicine, Philadelphia, Pennsylvania |
| **Shoudan Liang** | Neurobiology Department, Incyte Genomics, Inc., Palo Alto, California |
| **David J. Lockhart** | Laboratory of Genetics, The Salk Institute for Biological Studies, La Jolla, California |
| **Philippe Marc** | Laboratoire de Génétique Moléculaire, Centre National de la Recherche Scientifique UMR8541, ENS, Paris, France |
| **Robert Nadon** | Imaging Research, Inc. and Brock University, St. Catharines, Ontario, Canada |
| **Stanley F. Nelson** | Department of Human Genetics, UCLA School of Medicine, Los Angeles, California |
| **Siobhan Pickett** | Axon Instruments, Inc., Union City, California |
| **Marie-Claude Potier** | Neurobiologie et Diversité Cellulaire, Centre National de la Recherche Scientifique UMR7637, ESPCI, Paris, France |
| **Peter Ramm** | Imaging Research, Inc. and Brock University, St. Catharines, Ontario, Canada |
| **Nezar Rghei** | Imaging Research, Inc., St. Catharines, Ontario, Canada |

**Jean Rossier**   Neurobiologie et Diversité Cellulaire, Centre National de la Recherche Scientifique UMR7637, ESPCI, Paris, France

**Shishir Shah**   Spectral Genomics, Inc., Houston, Texas

**Soheil Shams**   BioDiscovery, Inc., Los Angeles, California

**Peide Shi**   Imaging Research, Inc., St. Catharines, Ontario, Canada

**Roland Somogyi**   Molecular Mining Corporation, Kingston, Ontario, Canada

**Edward Susko**   Dalhousie University, Halifax, Nova Scotia, Canada

**John Q. Trojanowski**   Center for Neurodegenerative Disease Research, Department of Pathology and Laboratory Medicine, University of Pennsylvania School of Medicine, Philadelphia, Pennsylvania

**Vivianna M. D. Van Deerlin**   Center for Neurodegenerative Disease Research, Department of Pathology and Laboratory Medicine, University of Pennsylvania School of Medicine, Philadelphia, Pennsylvania

**Damian Verdnik**   Axon Instruments, Inc., Union City, California

**David Wellis**   Axon Instruments, Inc., Union City, California

**Laurie W. Whitney**   Neuroimmunology Branch, National Institute of Neurological Disorders and Stroke, National Institutes of Health, Bethesda, Maryland

**Erik Woody**   University of Waterloo, Waterloo, Ontario, Canada

# Abbreviations

**AD**   Alzheimer's disease

**AMPA**   Alpha-amino-3-hydroxy-5-methyl-4-isoxazole-proprionic acid

**AMV-RT**   avian myeloblastosis reverse transcriptase

**ANOVA**   analysis of variance

**AO**   acridine orange

**APP**   amyloid precursor protein

**aRNA**   antisense RNA

**CCD**   charge-coupled device

**CNS**   central nervous system

**CV**   coefficient of variation

**dATP**   deoxyadenosine triphosphate

**dCTP**   deoxycytidine triphosphate

**DD**   differential display

**DEPC**   diethyl pyrocarbonate

**dntp**   deoxyribonucleoside triphosphate

**DRG**   dorsal root ganglia

**DTT**   dithiothreitol

**dUTP**   deoxyuridine triphosphate

**ES**   embryonic stem cells

**EST**   expressed sequence tag

**FDR**   false discovery rate

**G3PDH**   glucose-3-phosphate dehydrogenase

**GABA**   gamma-aminobutyric acid

**GADPH**   glyceraldehyde phosphate dehydrogenase

**GTP**   guanosine triphosphate

**HPRT**   hypoxanthine-guanine phosphoribosyl transferase

**5HT**   5-hydroxy-L-tryptophan

**IST**  in situ transcription

**IVT**  in vitro transcription

**kb**  kilobase (1000 base pairs)

**LCM**  laser capture microdissection

**MB**  megabase (1 million base pairs)

**MM**  mismatch

**MPCR**  multiplex polymerase chain reaction

**NA**  numerical aperture

**NBF**  neutral-buffered formalin

**NFT**  neurofibrillary tangle

**NGF**  nerve growth factor

**NIA**  National Institute on Aging

**PCA**  principal component analysis

**PCR**  polymerase chain reaction

**PET**  paraffin-embedded tissue

**PHFtau**  paired helical filament tau

**PM**  perfect match

**PMI**  postmortem interval

**PMT**  photomultiplier tube

**PNS**  peripheral nervous system

**QE**  quantum efficiency

**QTL**  quantitative trait loci

**RDA**  representational difference analysis

**RC**  resistor-capacitor

**RT**  reverse transcription

**SAGE**  serial analysis of gene expression

**SD**  standard deviation

**SDS**  sodium dodecylsulfate

**SNP**  single-nucleotide polymorphism

**SNR**  signal-to-noise ratio

**SPs**  senile plaques

**SSC**  sodium citrate

**SSH**  suppressive subtractive hybridization

**SSII**  SuperScript II

**STG**  superior temporal gyrus
**TSA**  tyramide substrate amplification
**TTP**  thymidine triphosphate
**UV**  ultraviolet
**VIP**  vasoactive intestinal peptide

# Index

Inferential analysis. *See* Statistical inference
Information, 273–274, 297–299. *See also* Data analysis; Web resources
array informatics and, 65–68
brain profiling and, 188–198
comparative analysis of microarrays, 275–277
explosion of, ix
gene prioritization, 277–282
management of, 66–68
pathway inference and, 282–287
reverse engineering and, 288–296
Shannon entropy and, 277–282
SNR and, 29–32
In silico methods, 111
In situ hybridization, xiv
brain tissue and, 204–206, 209, 213
candidate gene approach and, 226
gene expression analysis and, 224
large-scale expression and, 229
linear amplification and, 218, 222
oligonucleotides and, 177–179
In situ transcription, 204, 211, 221, 223
Insulin-like growth factor (IGF), 293
Intensity-based segmentation, 79–80
Intensity ratio, 87
Invitrogen, 18
In vitro methods, 111, 165–166, 258–259
Iterations, 63

Kainate, 239, 281, 290, 293–295
Klenow fragment, 221
K-means clustering, 286
Krox-24 element, 286
Kuhlmann, Sonia, 237–254, 312
Kuwahara filter, 74

Labeling, 2. *See also* Fluorescence
cDNA strategies and, 145–146, 152–155
microdissection and, 213–214
radioactive, 1, 10, 146–147, 151–153
specific expressions and, 167–170
Lambolez, Bertrand, 237–254, 312
Laminar variation, 212–213
Lasers, 11–13
beam diameter and, 36–37
dwell time and, 38
dye illumination and, 34–38

HeNe, 36
microdissection and, 215, 217
simultaneous scanning and, 40–41
spectral shifting and, 36
YAG, 36
LCM instruments, 217, 227
Least-squares method, 57
Le Bourdellès, Beatrice, 237–254, 313
Lee, Virginia M.-Y., 201–235, 313
Lenses, 38–39
Liang, Shoudan, 273–299, 313
Libraries. *See* Databases
Lid lifting, 9
Light
collection, 38–40
delivery, 34–38
excitation spectrum and, 35–36
Linear amplification, 217–223
Linear filters, 73
Line averaging, 47
Liver, 281
Lockhart, David J., 175–200, 313
Logarithms, 110–111
Low-throughput methods, 112

Macromolecules, 207
Majer Precision, Inc., 237
Mann-Whitney segmentation, 80–81, 92, 122–123
Mapping, 70–71, 274
Marc, Phillipe, 237–254, 313
Mass spectroscopy, 210
Mathematics. *See also* Data analysis; Statistical inference
Bonferroni procedure, 122, 138
default analysis algorithms, 183–184
digital conversion, 49–50
error, 112–132
least-squares method, 57
light delivery and, 34
linearity, 44
logarithms, 110–111
ratio calculation, 56–58
semiautomatic spotting algorithms, 76–77
Shannon entropy, 277–282
standard deviation (SD), 30, 89–90, 118–121, 129–133
Mean intensity, 86, 88–89